If Only My Doctor Had Told Me...

Your Rights as a Patient and the Law that Protects You

Written by
Meridith Berk

Copyright 2017 Meridith Berk

Old Town Publishing
OldTownPublishing.com

Table of Contents

Forward	7
Introduction	8

Informed Consent

The Legal Right that Could Save Your Life	10
A Brief History of Informed Consent	12
More About a Patient's Right to Give *Informed Consent*	14
What's My Diagnosis and How Did You Decide?	19
Tell Me More About the Recommended Treatment	28
What Alternatives Do I Have?	32
Acupuncture as a Recommended Treatment	38
Chiropractic Care as a Recognized Treatment Option	41
Massage as an Alternative Approach	43
Diet, Nutrition, and Exercise as Positive Health Care	44
The Alternative of Physical Therapy	46
Interview with an International Leader in Physical Therapy	48
Naturopathic Medicine as a Alternative	51
Traditional Chinese Medicine	53
Homeopathy as an Alternative	54
Ayurvedic Medicine	55

Mind-Body Therapies	56
Tai Chi - Another Well-Respected Alternative	57
Yoga is Another Popular Alternative	58
Interview with Noted Author and Yoga Instructor	60
Diagnoses Known to Respond Well to Alternatives	65
Special Note About Treatments for Pain	66
Special Note About Treatments for Emotional, Behavioral, and Mental Problems	71
Summary of the Alternative Step of Informed Consent	76
What if I Do Nothing?	78
How Much Information is Enough?	79
You May Need to Get a Second Opinion	83
Exceptions to the Law of Informed Consent	85
Barriers to Informed Consent	**88**
Fraudulent Practices and Physician Error	89
Industry Lobbying in Washington	89
Astroturfing as Marketing Plan and for Media Control	96
Pharmaceutical Advertising to Doctors	98

Conflicts of Interest	103
Pharmaceutical Advertising to Consumers (Drugs you don't need for diseases you don't have)	106
Time and Money	109
Doctor's Concern Over Offering Too Much Information	111
Patient's Failure to Know Their Rights	112
Patient's Inability to Understand	113
Lack of Patient Participation	114
Is the Doctor Unaware of Alternatives?	115
Become an Empowered Patient	117
If Only I'd Asked….	123

Appendix 127

Ethical Codes for the Medical Profession - The Road to Informed Consent

The Hippocratic Oath - Ancient and Modern
World Medical Association, Declaration of Geneva
World Medical Association International Code of Medical Ethics
Patient's Bill of Rights
Patients' Bill of Rights (AAPA)
Principles of Medical Ethics (AMA)
Basic Steps of Informed Consent

Charts Graphs and Images

Countries in Order of Lifespan
Countries Spending Most on Healthcare
Pharma Spending: Research vs. Marketing
Death by Medical Error

Interview with Donna Rybacki - Senior Care Specialist & Advocate

A Look at Informed Consent by Attorney, Tony Chicotel

A Patient's Rights Attorney Discusses Informed Consent

Glossary
Resources

Foreward

I have practiced law in California about 45 years and focused on issues about patients' rights in the mental field of psychiatry. Nothing is more important than the public realizing their role in the healthcare process and insisting that their medical advisors have great respect for the right of the patient to be informed and decide. I commend Meridith Berk for writing this book and urge all to read and apply it.

- Gary S. Brown
Patient's Rights Attorney

Introduction

The United States healthcare system is sick. We spend more money on our medical care than any other developed country, but our average life spans are shorter.

We take more drugs than other nations and pay far more for them. Three in five Americans take at least one prescription drug and nearly 15% take five or more prescription medications. Painkiller addiction has reached epidemic levels.

Accidental drug overdoses now kill more people each year than vehicle accidents. Prescription drug overdose occurs more frequently than overdoses from illicit drugs. Celebrities such as Michael Jackson, Heath Ledger and Prince, as well as the many thousands of people who never made a headline, have fallen prey to prescription drug addiction and death.

> *"Healthy citizens are the greatest asset any country can have."*
> *- Winston Churchill*

Medical errors are the third leading cause of death in America, right after heart disease and cancer.

Special interest groups have gained control of our medical system. As one of only two countries in the world that allow direct-to-consumer advertising by pharmaceutical companies, we in America are constantly barraged by advertisements marketing diseases and the drugs that treat them.

For doctors it's worse. Representatives from drug companies visit physicians at their offices and at hospitals bringing gifts and offering free lunches. In exchange, the doctor is required to listen to a sales pitch on the newest drugs manufactured by that pharmaceutical firm. As one drug company rep said, "The doctor thinks he's going to lunch with a friend, I know I'm buying lunch for a customer."

Major medical publications print articles many of which are nothing but drug marketing pieces dressed up as "medical research". Those articles and others are also surrounded by pharmaceutical advertisements.

How did our healthcare system get so out of control? How can we take back our medical care and return to thoughts of maintaining robust physical health rather than *managing* diseases and "disorders"?

I hope this book will help us take a step toward answering these questions and regaining power over our own medical choices and decisions.

Chapter 1
The Legal Right that Could Save Your Life

A powerful piece of legislation has been enacted in every state of the Union. If enforced, this one law could have an enormous effect on your medical care and even save your life.

This is the law of Informed Consent.

Unfortunately, no one ever told us about this law. Nowhere is it taught, posted, or explained. And it is vital to the health of each one of us.

The law of Informed Consent originates from the legal and ethical right the patient has to direct what happens to his or her body and from the ethical duty of the physician to involve the patient in his or her health care.

The most important goal is that the patient has an opportunity to be an active and informed participant in his or her health care decisions.

Every step of the law is designed to make sure doctors communicate with their patients in an informative and comprehensible way. This includes giving the individual a clear understanding of their diagnosis, the suggested treatment (including the risks involved), alternatives to the recommended treatment, and the possible outcome of having no treatment at all.

When I started working on this book, I asked people if they knew about this right of Informed Consent. No one I talked to had any idea this law existed and each had a story about a time they wished they'd known about this right - where they had a terrible reaction to a prescribed medication, had a relative who wished they hadn't undergone a surgery, or a friend who became innocently addicted to a medication and had to undergo serious withdrawals and rehabilitation in order to get his life back.

Nowhere in our education do we learn about our rights as patients - not in school, not from our parents, not from our doctors or nurses, not even from a PBS special. And, as patients, we do have rights. Ethical codes have long been established and doctors, to varying degrees, abide by these codes. However, we also have this important right that has been laid down in law - to determine what is done to our bodies in the course of medical care.

Informed Consent is the cornerstone of patient's rights and is at the heart of shared decision-making — the approach to medical treatment in which patients actively participate in their health care with their doctors.

It is a legal obligation due from a physician to his patient, an obligation that may only be met by the physician himself or herself talking directly with the patient. This obligation may not be delegated to any other medical or administrative staff.
It must be a live communication between physician and his or her patient, and not through use of consent forms, which are never a substitute for explanations and a real patient-doctor relationship.

Consent by the patient to any treatment must be voluntary, competent and informed. Consent is not considered valid if the patient does not understand the proposed treatment or has been misinformed.

Where other codes deal in ethical and moral principles, Informed Consent is a legally binding set of rules. *Informed Consent is a law*.

Chapter 2
A Brief History of Informed Consent

It took an extended series of lawsuits and court rulings, beginning in the early days of the 20th century, to bring about this law designed to protect a patient's simple right to be clearly informed and consulted in advance of any medical treatment or procedure.

The fight for participatory medicine began at the start of the nineteen-hundreds with the Supreme Court case involving a woman names Parmelia Davis whose surgeon removed her uterus and ovaries without having told her of his intentions.

The surgeon explained to the courts that he had deceived the patient so she would not refuse the operation. The surgeon's attorneys argued that unless the patient expressly forbids the act she consents to the doctor "performing such operation as in his best judgment is proper and essential to her welfare."

The Supreme Court disagreed, and in a 1905 opinion, declared that Americans' rights as free citizens prohibited "a physician or surgeon, however skillful or eminent…to violate without permission the bodily integrity of his patient…and [to operate] on him without his consent or knowledge."

In a 1914 Supreme Court decision in a similar case with a patient named Mary Schloendorff, Justice Benjamin Cardozo famously added, "A surgeon who performs an operation without his patient's consent commits an assault."

However, it was not until the late 1950s that patients acquired the right to be told not only what the doctor was going to do, but also the possible positive and negative effects of the treatment.

This requirement for "*Informed Consent*" resulted from a lawsuit filed by Martin Salgo, patient whose legs were left paralyzed following a hospital diagnostic procedure. Salgo claimed his doctors were legally liable for not having warned him of that risk.

The California Court of Appeals agreed, writing: *"A physician violates his duty to his patient and subjects himself to liability if he withholds any facts which are necessary to form the basis of an intelligent consent by the patient to the proposed treatment."*

That ruling was broadened in other cases over the next 15 years.

Finally, in 1972 a ruling came down from the US Court of Appeals requiring physicians to specifically disclose the risks in language the patient could actually understand. The decision involved a 19-year-old boy left paralyzed after a surgical procedure for back pain. The ruling made reference to an earlier Supreme Court declaration that "every human being of adult years and sound mind has a right to determine what shall be done with his own body."

In another important decision in 1972, the California Supreme Court declared that the "scope of the disclosure required of physicians defies simple definition" and must therefore "be measured by the patient's need, and *that need is whatever information is material to the decision.*"

This right to Informed Consent has continued to expand through ensuing decades until it has reached its current form.

Chapter 3
More About a Patient's Right to Give *Informed Consent*

Our ability as humans to reason, to choose, and to plan, helps raise us into the ranks of sentient beings. This is why respect for these characteristics remains closely linked to a respect for human dignity. Throughout the years, people have fought and died to defend human and patient rights and the right to Informed Consent that follows.

As most general practitioners will tell you, the practice of medicine works best as a team effort, a partnership between doctor and patient.

> As one primary care physician put it,
> *"Patient engagement is a wonder drug"*.

A doctor's recommendation is not law. We don't need to accept everything the doctor suggests or prescribes. In fact, more communication can help eliminate medical errors, reduce the cost of medical care, help increase the health and longevity of patients, and aid doctors in their own decision-making process.

By insisting on our right to Informed Consent we are moving away from the apparent comfort of simply obeying "doctor's orders" and stepping into a better level of medical care in which both patient and doctor actively participate in making the best medical decisions for that individual.

A failure in taking this right seriously has damaged the medical profession and the health of the very people it serves.

Reinstituting this right to Informed Consent in every doctor's visit and every physician-patient interchange will put back that level of communication and trust that is at the very heart of medical practice.

Here is a statement about Informed Consent from the National Library of Medicine

"Informed Consent is a legal obligation due from a physician to his patient, an obligation which may not be met by the physician's skillful treatment of his patient. It may only be met by the treating physician obtaining from his patient knowing authorization for carrying out the intended medical procedure. The physician is required to disclose whatever would be material to his patient's decision, including the nature and purpose of the procedure, and the risks and alternatives. The disclosures should be made by the physician to his patient, and not through use of consent forms which are not particular to individual patients."

Also from the National Library of Medicine

"In health care, Informed Consent refers to the process whereby the patient and the health care practitioner engage in a dialogue about a proposed medical treatment's nature, consequences, harms, benefits, risks, and alternatives. Informed Consent is a fundamental principle of health care.

The process of Informed Consent can be considered a patient safety issue from several perspectives. At the extreme, performing a procedure on a patient without his or her consent has been considered by the courts to be a form of battery.

Informed Consent may also be indirectly related to patient safety in that, when done well, it opens a dialogue between the patient and provider so that the patient can ask questions, knows what to expect during and after procedure, and can, at least theoretically, help to avert medical errors. If doctors have to explain the thinking behind their recommended treatments and the potential effects, they might be more cautious.

It should be self-evident that a physician's adherence to the doctrine of Informed Consent requires the physician to disclose enough about the risks and benefits of proposed treatments that the patient becomes sufficiently informed to participate in shared decision-making.

In general, studies have shown improved patient outcomes with effective physician-patient communication and increased patient empowerment. Patient education has also been associated with preventing medical errors."

> ***"If doctors have to explain the thinking behind their recommended treatments and the potential effect, they might be more cautious."***
> ***- National Library of Medicine***

The basic pillar on which Informed Consent rests is the right of any individual to determine and agree to what is done to his or her body. But consent cannot be considered truly given if the patient doesn't understand what the treatment is all about and what other choices exist. The doctor must be sure the patient understands and can give not just consent, but Informed Consent to any treatment. This is what the steps of Informed Consent are all about.

If a doctor fails to obtain Informed Consent from a patient this can be considered negligence or even battery. Courts have differed over various interpretations of the law, but the point here is that it is a law and one that you have a right to insist is applied to you.

Not all diagnoses and their treatments require long conversations about options and alternatives. A cut requires stitches, and a broken bone needs to be set in order to heal correctly. However, for anything more complex or with treatments that come with significant risks a full application of Informed Consent is both an ethical and legal requirement.

Basic Features of Everyday Informed Consent

Informed Consent is the process by which the treating health care provider (not a nurse, administrator, or pharmacist) discloses appropriate information to a competent patient or their advocate so that the patient may make an educated, voluntary choice to accept or refuse treatment.

The Law Regarding Informed Consent Requires the Physician (not a Delegated Representative) Disclose and Discuss With the Patient the Following:

* The diagnosis, if known

* The nature and purpose of a proposed treatment or procedure

* The risks and benefits of proposed treatment or procedure

* Alternatives (regardless of costs or extent covered by insurance)

* The risks and benefits of alternatives

* The risks and benefits of not receiving treatments or undergoing procedures

Source: American Medical Association

A patient often feels vulnerable, anxious, and powerless in a stressful medical situation. Doctors need to understand this and not take advantage of the situation to push across their view. To encourage the voluntary participation of the patient, the physician must make it clear that the individual is expected to play a role in the decision-making process.

As part of the Informed Consent process, the doctor is required to share the reasons behind any diagnosis or recommended treatment with the patient.

The full understanding of the situation and the treatment recommendation and alternatives by the patient is at the core of Informed Consent. This is why doctors must be able to explain each step of Informed Consent in layperson's terms. The information provided is useless if the patient can't understand it. The doctor should check the patient's understanding along the way.

> *"A patient has the right to be informed about their medical condition, the risks and benefits of treatment and appropriate alternatives."*
> *- The Law of Informed Consent*

Chapter 4
What's My Diagnosis and How Did You Decide?

Proper diagnosis lies at the heart of any medical system and is the first step of Informed Consent. You go to the doctor with a physical ailment and you want to know what it is. Is it serious? What can be done about it? Medical names for illnesses and diseases are usually derived from Latin or sometimes named for the person who discovered them. These terms are seldom part of everyday language. This holds true for the more modern psychiatric "disorders", such as ADHD, OCD, manic-depressive, etc.

When you ask your doctor for your diagnosis, write it down. Get help with the spelling as needed. Then, get him or her to explain it to you in plain English.

This first step is vital. It ensures you and your physician start out your discussion on the same page.

The practice of medicine, as with many other professions, involves plenty of jargon. This special language becomes so commonplace among practitioners that they often forget these specialized terms are meaningless to others.

> *"You must learn to talk clearly. The*
> *jargon of scientific terminology which*
> *rolls off your tongues is mental garbage"*
> *- Martin H. Fischer*
> *Physician and Teacher*

It does you no good to be told you have onychomycosis. Most patients would have no idea what the word means or whether this is a deadly or frightening condition or one that could be ignored. However, when the doctor tells the person that what they have is a fungal infection of one or more of their nails, this makes more sense and a real communication and discussion of options can occur.

Before you can expect a sensible and workable treatment, an accurate diagnosis must be found. The patient needs to know the nature and scope of his or her diagnosis, not just a name or label. And sometimes the doctor just doesn't know. It would be nice if our doctors knew everything about the body and every possible medical problem, but they don't.

This is especially true when it comes to psychiatric labels and emotional and mood problems, where there are no accurate methods of determining their existence and current medical treatments are dangerous and uncertain.

Don't Accept Every Diagnosis You're Given

The pharmaceutical industry working in conjunction with the American Psychiatric Association has managed to turn many honest human emotions, behaviors, and even personality traits into "disorders" and "diseases". This has been helped along in no small measure by very well planned advertising campaigns labeled by pharmaceutical marketer Vince Perry as "Branding a Condition".

"Many a small thing has been made large by the right kind of advertising"
- Mark Twain

Professor of psychiatry, Thomas Szasz calls this "The Medicalization of Everyday Life." In his book of that title Dr. Szasz describes in detail how conditions become "medicalized" and are then open to "treatment".

He goes on to explain how discovering a disease is not the same as creating a diagnosis. Depression is not the same as malaria. There are times when being depressed is an appropriate emotion. It is never appropriate to have malaria.

The quest for new conditions to diagnose and new diseases to create does not stop at mental states. Anyone would have thought there were plenty of diseases is this world, but apparently much of the pharmaceutical industry does not agree.

This powerful industry works tirelessly to invent new illnesses and convince us we are suffering from them.

This is known as "disease mongering", a name introduced by health and science writer Lynn Payer in her 1992 book *Disease-Mongers: How Doctors, Drug Companies, and Insurers Are Making You Feel Sick.*

Payer defined disease mongering as *"trying to convince essentially well people that they are sick, or slightly sick people that they are very ill."*

Ray Moynihan, Iona Heath and David Henry in an article for the *British Medical Journal referred to this as* "the corporate construction of disease". "There's a lot of money to be made from telling healthy people they're sick." "Pharmaceutical companies are actively involved in sponsoring the definition of diseases and promoting them to both prescribers and consumers."

> ***The fundamental trick in disease mongering is to inflate a common every day condition, graduating it from a nuisance into a disease, illness, or disorder requiring immediate attention.***

Lynn Payer identified many disease-mongering tactics. Among them are:

• Taking a normal function and implying that there's something wrong with it and that it should be treated

• Taking a common symptom that could mean anything and making it sound as if it is a sign of a serious disease

- Describing suffering that isn't necessarily there, but planting it in the public's conscious as something to worry about

- Defining as large a proportion of the population as possible as suffering from the "disease"

- Defining a condition as an indication of a disease, as a deficiency disease or as a chemical or hormonal imbalance

- Recruiting doctors to spin the message and consistently pounding their message to doctors through journal articles, drug reps, "thought leaders", continuing education seminars, and advertising.

- Using statistics selectively to exaggerate the benefits of treatment

- Promoting the treatment as risk free (hiding or negating the risks)

Healthcare watchdogs have been trying to stop this cycle of selling a disease and then offering the "cure". They have, for example, identified several "illnesses" as examples of *disease mongering*. They are not saying these conditions don't exist at all. The ailments do bother some people, some of the time. But the extent to which they occur in our society and the
degree to which they hamper people's lives are wildly exaggerated - and all in the pursuit of profits.

Among these "illnesses" and "disorders" are Attention Deficit Hyperactivity Disorder (ADHD), bipolar disorder, depression (as a disease to be labeled and drugged, as opposed to feeling sad, down, depressed, apathetic, etc., which would require an entirely different solution - on none at all), erectile dysfunction, female sexual dysfunction, bipolar disorder, restless legs syndrome, osteoporosis, social shyness (also called social anxiety disorder and social phobia), irritable bowel syndrome and balding.

A note on ADHD in the United States:

Children in the United States are diagnosed with ADHD at an alarming rate, far more frequently than they are in other developed countries, such as France. In the U.S., as least 9% of school-aged children have been diagnosed with ADHD and have been put on pharmaceutical medications. In France, only 0.5% of their children are diagnosed with ADHD and put on drugs. The French prefer to look for the underlying issue causing the behavioral problems and to address those with counseling, as opposed to using the pharmaceutical Band-Aid to mask the symptoms. Considering the frightening potential side effects of ADHD medications, the French may be onto something here.

The diagnosis of ADHD for children and adults continues to soar with the ever-expanding set of criteria for the labeling of this "disorder". With the diagnoses come the concurrent increase in prescribing of psychotropic medications to control the behavior (which many educators and doctors feel is a normal activity level) associated with this "disorder". The United States is the consumer of over 85% of the world's supply of methylphenidate, a controlled Schedule II narcotic. This is despite the fact that originally consensus of opinion was that a powerful psychotropic medication such as methylphenidate (known under brand names Ritalin, Concerta, and others) should only be used in the most severe cases, and only after safer treatment alternatives have been tried and proven ineffective.

A controlled Schedule II narcotic is a drug deemed to have great potential for addiction, abuse, and diversion into illegal drug trade. This is why these drugs are designated controlled substances and are stringently regulated on an international level.

Some of the effects these drugs can cause include:
nervousness
restlessness
chest pain
depression
hallucinations

seizures
difficulty falling asleep
difficulty staying asleep
aggressive or hostile behavior
unusual changes in personality

(These are just a few, dozens more are listed on the government website listed in the back of this book.)

A report out of DePaul University Libraries from Spring of 2014 written by Rita Barnett Rose explains that, not only could the prescribing of this type of medication be considered morally reprehensible, especially when the decision is being made by someone other than the person taking the medication, such as a child, it's being prescribed for a mental health "disorder" the very authenticity of which has been, for decades, under debate.

According to the same report in the DePaul Journal of Health Care Law, "The use of psychotropic medication to treat any presumed mental health disorder always involves the risk of serious harm."

Whatever your opinion about the validity of ADHD as a mental illness, it just makes sense that you make absolutely sure you are given full Informed Consent about the treatment your doctor recommends, including drug side effects and risks, and that you are told the alternatives. And as always, if you feel you are not being given all the information you need, get a second opinion.

I have a difficult time imagining we are so much more in need of heavy medication here in the United States than people in other countries. Perhaps we are just a nation of the over-diagnosed.

Considering the problem with addiction and drug abuse we are currently fighting here in the U.S., it seems only sensible to avoid medication when possible and search for alternatives that are less intrinsically harmful and more focused on long term health.

Just a moment ago I ran across another example of *disease mongering.* The evil genius of marketing has raised the common irritation of having dry eyes to the level of a disease, hereinafter to be known as Chronic Dry Eye Disease (CDED).

Oddly enough, at least two drugs are available to treat this terrible problem. In one advertisement, we are instructed to, "ask your doctor about Xiidra", a drug that just came out a little over two months ago. Meanwhile, the manufacturer of Restasis, another dry eye drug, got a patent extension to keep away generic drug manufacturers until 2024. Their ads, naturally, tell us to ask about Restasis.

Now, I know that some people certainly suffer from the discomfort of dry eyes. A year or so ago my dry eyes were driving me mad. When I went to the ophthalmologist he was smart enough to ask me what I did for a living. When I told him I was in front of my computer writing, researching, and looking at cat videos 12 hours a day, he gave me a simple solution, which worked for me. The doctor said to look away from the computer screen every half hour or so, cover my eyes with my cupped palms, and blink rapidly for a minute or so. It turns out, when we look at a computer don't blink as frequently as we normally do. This causes our eyes to become dry. The simple solution is to blink more.

Other causes of having dry eyes, will require other solutions, but is having dry eyes really a disease? Underlying diseases can have dry eyes as one of their symptoms and some medications list dry eyes as a side effect. In these cases, you'd want to make sure you're addressing the cause, not just covering it up with eye drops.

Since we're on the subject of diagnosis, some diseases associated with dry eyes include vitamin A deficiency, autoimmune/connective tissue disease, hepatitis C infection, HIV infection, Sjögren's syndrome, diabetes mellitus, and some hormone deficiencies.

Some medications, such as antihistamines, antidepressants, beta-blockers, diuretics, some chemotherapy drugs, and oral contraceptives, may decrease tear production.

Certain occupational and environmental factors can increase the likelihood of someone having dry eyes. These include; living in a low humidity area, high room temperature, wind exposure, pollution and poor air quality, smoking, and decreased blink rates due to sustained computer use or reading.

A diet low in omega-3 fatty acids or one too high in omega-6 fatty acids can affect the dryness of our eyes as well.

Sorting out the reasons for a condition, such as this, is real diagnosis. It's what doctors are supposed to do and not the job of advertising. Although it's a lot to ask, we all need to ignore pharmaceutical advertising and resist the temptation to ask our doctors about the latest in drugs and diseases.

But, these commercials are designed to give people who are just fine, yet another disease to worry about. The manufacturer's ads are also designed to get the person to make sure they leave the doctor's office with that prescription.

Disease mongering affects us all. A huge psychological burden is placed upon us when we are told to think of ourselves as diseased when we are not.

And there are the financial costs, affecting us both personally and as members of the greater society in which we live.

Treating these "illnesses" with pharmaceuticals is expensive and no tax-funded healthcare system, such as Medicare or care for our veterans can sustain the cost of all these new diseases and the drugs to treat them.

Unfortunately, with near limitless profits to be made from both legitimate sales of medical drugs and from those sold as part of disease mongering, pharmaceutical companies are rich, very rich, and extremely powerful.

More on how "Big Pharma" creates barriers to Informed Consent later. Meanwhile, just know there's lots of money behind convincing you and your doctor that you need a pill for every possible complaint.

Knowing this, we can at least try to outsmart the efforts of the disease mongers to pathologize every moment, every feeling, every experience of our existence

Naming is not the same as *diagnosing. Advertising a condition does not make it a disease.*

You can also do yourself and your doctor a favor by ignoring, as much as you possibly can, all the advertisements for diseases and the drugs that cure them.

It can help if you understand what's going on and how these advertising campaigns work. (This process is covered later in this book.)

Meanwhile, ignoring the lure of advertisements, you will want to know how the doctor came by the diagnosis. You'll want to be told what tests were performed and you'll want to know what those tests revealed. What *physical* condition or situation did the doctor observe? The less exact the diagnosis, the more you should think in terms of getting a second opinion.

A true and honest diagnosis that is based on accurate and measurable data is the first step in the law of Informed Consent and the starting point for any workable treatment or solution.

Chapter 5
Tell Me More About The Treatment You're Recommending Including Risks and Benefits

Risks and the Probability of Success

The next step, after a full discussion of your diagnosis, is for the physician to tell you about the benefits, risks, and potential harm of a proposed treatment or procedure. These must be explained no matter the recommended treatment.

Any prescribing physician has a duty to warn their patients of the risks and complications connected with any prescribed medication. Having these risks explained by a piece or paper, a nurse, or a pharmacist is not sufficient to fulfill the responsibility of Informed Consent.

Physicians are sometimes reluctant to give all the information about a drug or other treatment for fear of frightening the patient away from consenting. But that's the point of Informed Consent. The patient needs all the information to make an intelligent decision. If the patient is frightened away from a particular treatment, it may force the physician to find a safer solution.

Some questions that need to be answered are: "What is the probability of success using the proposed treatment or procedure? "What results can I realistically expect?"

If the treatment is a medication, "How long will I need to take this medication?" "Is this drug addictive and does it have any long term side effects?" "What is the likely outcome if I don't take it at all?"

You should also ask how long the prescribed medication has been on the market. Find out why this medication is being prescribed over a different, possibly cheaper, older, more tested medication. Does the doctor have a relationship with the drug manufacturer and does he or she accept lunches or gifts from representatives from that company?

Questions continue to arise regarding how much information patients need about the risks and benefits of treatment. The ultimate test is whether the individual has sufficient information to make an informed decision regarding whether to consent to treatment or not.

If, due to the risks involved with the proposed treatment, the patient doesn't want to do it, the doctor also has the other steps of Informed Consent to fall back on - the alternatives.

It's as much up to the patient to make sure they understand these risks as it is for the doctor to explain them. If, by some chance, the patient becomes addicted or suffers damage by taking a prescribed drug or undergoing a procedure, it's not the FDA or the physician that suffers, it's the patient and his or her family.

There is no medical magic wand and far too frequently the treatments that have been recommended turn out to have risks that outweigh the possible benefits.

What must be disclosed?

All material risks must be disclosed. A material risk is one that might cause a reasonable patient to decide not to undergo the recommended treatment.

The magnitude of the risk is part of the decision whether or not the risk need be revealed. For example, a 1 in 10,000 risk of death would always be disclosed. However 1 in 10,000 risk of a mild and fleeting headache does not need to be brought up.

Hidden or Understated Side Effects of Prescription Medication

As prescription drug use continues to rise at an alarming pace (3 in 5 Americans takes at least 1 prescription drug) and addiction continues to destroy lives, it becomes imperative that doctors give fair warning about all the medications they prescribe.

Prescribing physicians have a primary duty to warn patients about the risks and complications of prescribed medications.

Patients and doctors both suffer when warnings and side effects connected with a prescription are somehow hidden from view.

Drug companies try to underplay side effects in their communications to doctors and doctors don't seem all that anxious to relate these to their patients.

> *"Half the modern drugs could well*
> *be thrown out the window except*
> *that the birds might eat them.*
> *- Martin H. Fischer*
> *Physician and Teacher*

I was in my doctor's office, browsing through magazines the other day and ran across an article about the treatment of diabetic neuropathy. The article included a table containing what the writer called, "Common medications in the treatment of peripheral neuropathy". These treatments included many drugs with serious side effects and Black Box Warnings such as amitryptaline, desipramine, and venlafaxine. However, the writer of the article only included three or four "Adverse Events" for these drugs and no side effects.

A busy doctor could go down the list and prescribe one of these medications. Some doctors may do so without thinking about side effects, warnings, and contra-indications attributable to these drugs. Doctors are busy people. They get a great deal of their information from pharmaceutical reps and ads in medical publications. In order to keep the articles brief authors use abbreviated lists of side effects, "adverse events" and other warnings, thereby wittingly or unwittingly playing into the hands of the pharmaceutical companies. The bottom line is that publications underplay the side affects and promote the advantages.

Let's take the drug amitryptaline. In the table accompanying the article the adverse events listed for this drug are "anticholineric, weight gain, arrhythmias". In actual fact the FDA Adverse Events Reporting System (AERS) includes more than 1,500 individually reported adverse events connected with this drug, including delirium, depression, blindness and death.

The side effects and warnings include, *"new or worsening depression, thinking about harming or killing yourself or planning on doing so, extreme worry, agitation, panic attacks, difficulty falling asleep or staying asleep, aggressive behavior, irritability, acting without thinking, severe restlessness, and frenzied abnormal excitement"* - From FDA Black Box Warnings for amitryptaline

Additional side effects for this drug are: *crushing chest pain, nausea, vomiting, dizziness, fainting, hallucinating, and seizures.*

The writer of that article about treating diabetic neuropathy did a great disservice to the doctors who might rely on the abbreviated information given in the article and the patients of those doctors.

Doctors and patients both need full disclosure of the dangers attached to taking pharmaceutical products. Perhaps they would then seek out treatments that offer the best benefits with the least amount of risk.

And just because a doctor has not personally observed a side effect or heard a complaint from one of their patients doesn't mean it doesn't happen.

Treatments such as surgery and medication save lives and help many, many people. However, Informed Consent insists the doctor and patient talk things over and come up with the best, most risk-free treatments. Real and interested communication is the key to patients receiving the health care that's best for them. Every doctor's appointment doesn't need to end with a handshake and a prescription.

Chapter 6
What Alternatives Do I Have?
Alternatives (regardless of costs or extent covered by insurance)

The Risks and Benefits of Alternatives

The law of Informed Consent includes the obligation doctors have to inform their patients of alternative treatments. First, of course, doctors will need to inform *themselves* of the available, workable alternatives. Some of these are used successfully overseas and need to become better known in the United States.

Part of the appeal of alternative medicine and the use of health foods, supplements, diet, and exercise is that this kind of therapy leaves people in control of their own health. Additionally, these do not involve the placement of a label of having a disease or 'disorder'.

If you are stressed, burnt out, exhausted, or anxious (something we all are from time to time) you can get acupuncture, go on walks with a friend, take valerian root or St. John's Wort. To be prescribed Prozac or another psychotropic medication, you first have to be given a mental illness. And as is covered elsewhere, pharmaceutical companies have spent millions convincing us we all have one or more illnesses and should take drugs as opposed to engaging in lifestyle changes.

Here is a quote from the American Family Physician magazine from the article, Appropriate Prescribing of Medications: An Eight-Step Approach

"Nonpharmacologic therapy remains an important treatment option. The woman with diabetes and the added diagnosis of hypertension may not need medication if she loses weight and exercises. A patient with chronic headaches may respond to relaxation training, and a patient with insomnia may improve with better sleep hygiene.

Studies have shown that physicians often write prescriptions of doubtful benefit because of perceived pressure to prescribe medications. However, these perceptions may be inaccurate. Asking a patient directly about therapeutic goals may shed light on his or her willingness to use nonpharmacologic options when available."

> *"Some day when you have time,*
> *look into the business of prayer,*
> *amulets, baths, and poultices,*
> *and discover much valuable therapy*
> *the profession has cast on the dump."*
> *- Martin H. Fischer*
> **Physician and Teacher**

Despite the fact that most complementary or alternative medicine is not covered by insurance and patients have to pay all costs out of their own pockets, nearly 40% of adults report using some kind of alternative treatment. This willingness to pay out of their own pockets reflects the public's general acceptance of Complementary and Alternative Medicine (CAM) and also suggests that CAM therapies have benefits that outweigh their costs.

Over a third of Americans seek help for their health in a place that is outside their doctor's office.

Many times, doctors aren't even aware their patients are taking supplements, seeing a chiropractor, or doing whatever mental or spiritual healing works for them. The patients, afraid they'll appear stupid or will be told to stop, don't mention these to their doctors.

This is another indication that doctors must improve the level of communication they have with their patients and take the time to ensure real Informed Consent takes place.

This also shows that doctors need to spend a little time learning about alternatives, their benefits and risks. How else will they be able to inform their patients? This doesn't mean a trained physician needs to know every product, service or therapy that results from an Internet search or shows up on daytime television.

Complementary and alternative medicine has become part of our culture and our healthcare. Until medical schools in the United States add more complementary and alternative medical approaches to their curriculum it will have to be up to the individual physician to educate himself or herself on widely accepted Complementary and Alternative Medicine (CAM) approaches.

When a patient, an advocate, or legal surrogate, specifically asks about alternative treatment options, a physician must provide this information, even if he or she does not agree such alternatives are effective. The doctor may not impose his or her values on his or her patients or substitute their own fears or other considerations for those of their patients. Only with full communication of the material information called for in Informed Consent can true doctor and patient collaboration toward the best patient health outcome be expected.

Just because a doctor hasn't been trained in another health specialty or type of treatment and is not familiar with it doesn't mean that it doesn't work. Don't accept a doctor telling you not to try an alternative solution just because he doesn't understand it.

It's time for physicians to embrace alternatives and the part these can play in their patients' health.

Complementary and Alternative Medicine (CAM) is defined as a group of diverse medical and health care systems, practices, and products that are not presently considered to be part of conventional medicine.

If patients are aware of these alternatives, why aren't more doctors?

The chiropractic association or naturopathic doctors, yoga instructors, nutritionists or exercise coaches don't have the power and money to put their information in front of medical doctors in the same way drug companies do. Doctors are inundated with information (accurate and false) in their journals, continuing education programs, and in visits from the drug company representatives that haunt the waiting rooms of medical offices.

And doctors have a great deal of information to keep up with. New drugs and other forms of treatment become available on a regular basis.

With all the calls upon their time, patients to see, reports to write, articles and journals to keep up with, it's understandable that medical doctors don't have or want to take the time to learn about *all* the alternative and complementary treatments available and the risks and benefits of these. No sensible person could expect this.

However, there are quite a few complementary and alternative treatment options that have made their way into the mainstream of our healthcare system and these should be known well enough for the practitioner to advise a patient on the possible applicability of any one or more of these to his or her diagnosed condition.

In fact, many doctors are happy to have additional treatments available for their patients when the usual protocol fails to work or comes with too many risks.

On some lists (even one provided by the U.S. Center for Disease Control (CDC)), exercise, nutrition and diet are placed in the category of complementary and alternative treatments.

These used to be among the first treatments suggested by physicians to treat many conditions and concerns.

Per the law of Informed Consent, medical doctors must provide their patients with information on alternative treatments for their condition. So, obviously it's expected that they will become at least marginally aware of the alternatives available to patients.

Once again, we are not asking doctors to step out from under the umbrella of conventional medicine and accepted Western medical treatments when we suggest they inform their patients about alternatives. Not only is this part of the Informed Consent law, the U.S. Department of Health and Human Services has an entire division, the National Center for Complementary and Integrative Medicine, dedicated to this area of healing.

Traditional Western medical hospitals and organizations endorse, and recommend many different alternative therapies. For instance, the Mayo Clinic, suggest the use of Tai Chi and Yoga in the treatment of Rheumatoid Arthritis.

The City of Hope is currently researching the use of Superfoods in the treatment of cancer. Memorial Sloan Kettering, another top cancer hospital in the U.S. offers integrative medical services, designed to work with traditional medical treatments. These alternatives include massage therapy, acupuncture, yoga, music, dance therapy and martial arts.

The Mayo Clinic, which tied for #1 on the US News and World Report list of Best Hospitals in the US for 2015 has published a series of books offering advice on alternative treatments for conditions from chronic pain to heart health, diabetes and Alzheimer's.

Another top ranked American hospital, Johns Hopkins, devotes an entire section of its website to Complementary and Alternative Medical therapies.

We can see that medical specialists at the top of their profession are aware of the potential benefits of alternative therapies and educate the public about them. Physicians in general practice need to follow this example.

An additional sign of the general acceptance of complementary and alternative medicine (CAM), is that sometimes patients can receive insurance coverage for CAM health care expenses by obtaining a prescription for these services from their primary physician. This prescription must include the diagnosis, as well as frequency and length of the necessary treatment. While this measure will not guarantee coverage, many insurance providers will approve all doctor-approved physicians. The most commonly approved services include chiropractic care, massage therapy, physical therapy, and homeopathy.

You can see that patients, hospitals, and insurance providers are aware of a huge number of effective alternative therapies. It's time doctors made themselves aware of these alternative treatment options too.

This is taken directly from the National Institute of Health
"A distinct trend toward the integration of complementary and alternative medicine (CAM) therapies with the practice of conventional medicine is occurring. Hospitals are offering CAM therapies, health maintenance organizations (HMOs) are covering such therapies, a growing number of physicians use CAM therapies in their practices, insurance coverage for CAM therapies is increasing, and integrative medicine centers and clinics are being established, many with close ties to medical schools and teaching hospitals."

Here are some of the alternative and complementary therapies used by the American public, and practiced by or recommended by major hospitals and insurance companies.

These practices are listed here because you may need to educate your doctor on alternatives.

As I mentioned before, despite the clarity of the law, many doctors don't offer alternatives or even credit ones the patient may be using. So, it's up to us to change our healthcare by educating our doctors.

Chapter 7
Acupuncture as a Recommended Treatment

Acupuncture is one of the oldest and most commonly used medical procedures in the world.

This traditional form of Chinese medicine is designed to balance the energy flows within the body by stimulating specific points, known as acupoints.

During a typical acupuncture treatment 5 to 20 fine needles are inserted into the patient's body at various depths. Needles are typically left in for less than 1 hour. Acupuncturists may increase the stimulation by manipulating the needles (periodically twirling the needles) or by applying heat or electrical stimulation to the needles. An alternative technique includes using laser rather than needles to stimulate acupoints.

The medical practice of acupuncture is based on the premise that a form of energy called "qi" travels along prescribed pathways within the body. This theory proposes that "qi" is responsible for maintaining good health by providing internal stability through the regulation of vital body function. Excess or deficiency in the flow of this energy is thought to result in disease. Stimulation of specific acupoints along the body's pathways can restore balance and return the individual to health.

Acupuncture has been practiced in Asia for more than 4,000 years. The practice spread to Korea and Japan in the 6th century AD. By the 19th century AD the medical practice of acupuncture had been introduced to Europe, Australia and North America.

In the United States, more than 3 million adults undergo treatment each year. With increasing evidence to support its practice, acupuncture has been integrated within many hospitals around the world. In the U.S., acupuncture likely to
be covered by insurance.

In the United Kingdom (UK), acupuncture has been made available within the National Health Service (NHS) through physiotherapists, pain clinics and primary care clinics.

A scientific study conducted by the World Health Organization in 2003 indentified numerous conditions positively affected by acupuncture treatments. A full breakdown of this analysis makes interesting reading and is referenced on the website refernced book in the resources section under "Alternatives.

The list is long and has been edited for this book to remove unusual medical conditions and those terms with which we, as patients, would be unlikely to be familiar.

Acupuncture has shown to be a successful treatment for:

Abdominal pain
Acne
Adverse reactions to radiotherapy and/or chemotherapy
Anxiety
Asthma
Bell's Palsy
Cancer pain
Cardiac neurosis
Depression
Dermatitis
Diabetes mellitus, non-insulin-dependent
Earache
Female infertility
Fibromyalgia
Gout (a type of arthritis)
Hay Fever
Hot flashes
Indigestion
Headache
Hypertension (high blood pressure)
Hypotension (low blood pressure)
Insomnia
Jaw pain
Knee pain

Labor pain
Leukopenia (decrease in the number of white blood cells)
Low back pain
Menstrual cramps
Morning sickness
Nausea and vomiting
Neck pain
Obesity
Opium, cocaine and heroin dependence
Osteoarthritis of the knee or hip
PMS
Postoperative pain (pain after surgery)
Renal colic (painful kidney stone)
Rheumatoid arthritis
Schizophrenia
Sciatica
Shingles
Shoulder pain and stiffness
Sore throat (including tonsillitis)
Spine pain, acute
Sprain
Stiff neck
Stress
Stroke
Tennis elbow
Tourette syndrome
Ulcerative colitis (chronic disease of the large intestine sometimes called IBD)
Urinary-tract infection (recurrent)
Whooping cough

Risks Associated with Acupuncture

Per the Mayo Clinic, risks associated with acupuncture are few and include: soreness, infections (if needles are reused), and organ damage (if needles put In too deep). These last two can be avoided by using a licensed and competent acupuncturist.
Patients with bleeding disorders, who are pregnant, or have a pacemaker, may not be good candidates for acupuncture.

Chapter 8
Chiropractic Care as a Recognized Treatment Option

In recent decades chiropractic treatment has grown in popularity and medical recognition.

The chiropractic profession is concerned with the prevention, diagnosis, and treatment of disorders related to the neuromusculoskeletal system (system of nerves, muscles, bones, and joints) and the effects it has on the patient's general physical health. The application of chiropractic techniques emphasizes manual manipulation and joint adjustment with particular emphasis on restoring function.

Based on the chiropractic approach, the body is regarded as a neuromusculoskeletal system in which disorder in one part of the system disturbs the other parts. Therefore, disorders in the body structure are removed so that stresses on the body's nervous system can be alleviated and the general health of the body can be restored.

Some chiropractors also offer nutritional and lifestyle counseling.

The practice of chiropractic was founded by Daniel David Palmer in the United States in 1895, and gradually attracted its proponents among doctors and other healers. Chiropractic is now practiced worldwide.

The primary reasons patients seek chiropractic care are back pain, pain in neck, shoulders, extremities, and pain from arthritis and headaches (including migraines). Other common reasons people visit a chiropractor include PMS, digestive problems and respiratory ailments.

Chiropractic treatments have also proven effective on many other conditions, including:

Anxiety
Cancer and cancer treatment related pain
Disc disorders in the spine and neck
Fibromyalgia
Flexibility and range of motion difficulties
Headaches (including migraine and tension headaches)
Immune system problems
Jaw pain and problems (TMJ)
Lumbar stenosis (narrowing of the spinal canal)
Neck pain
Pinched nerve in the neck and lower back
Repetitive strain injuries
Sacroiliac joint pain
Shoulder pain
Sports injuries
Sprains and strains
Stress
Whiplash

Integration of Chiropractic Care with Mainstream Medicine

Chiropractic services are now largely or fully integrated with medical and other mainstream health care services in a number of countries. In the US chiropractic services are now available in the military and veterans' administration hospital and health care systems, and through Harvard University's health care network. Harvard Medical School and Brigham and Women's Hospital both utilize the use of chiropractic care as an adjunct to conventional medical treatments.

In the words of Wayne Jonas, MD, Founding Director, Office of Alternative Medicine, US National Institutes of Health:

"The chiropractic profession is assuming its valuable and appropriate role in the health care system in this country and around the world. As this happens the professional battles of the past will fade and the patient at last will be the true winner."

Chapter 9
Massage as an Alternative Health Care Approach

Manipulation and massage therapy, including Swedish massage, Thai massage, deep tissue massage and sports massage help reduce pain, stress, and muscle tension.

These may also be helpful in relieving anxiety, improving digestive problems, helping with soft tissue strains, and alleviating headaches.

When used as a complement to cancer treatment, oncology massage helps improve the patient's quality of life. These benefits include improved relaxation, sleep, and immune function, as well as relief of fatigue, nausea, anxiety and pain.

Chapter 10
Diet / Nutrition / Supplements / Superfoods and Exercise (oddly considered alternative or complementary)

The World Health Organization estimates that 80 percent of the world's population in the world use traditional medicines made up of natural products like herbs, vitamins, minerals, probiotics, melatonin, fish oil, and others in hopes of enhancing their health and wellbeing.

Superfoods: The term "superfood" refers to anything you eat that contains large amounts of antioxidants, fiber, vitamins, minerals, and polyphenols. Adding these foods to your diet is thought to reduce the risk of certain chronic diseases, to boost the immune system and to prolong life.

This is another area of complementary and alternative medicine that is acknowledged as effective by what I would call the *western medical establishment*.

In fact, researchers at the City of Hope have found five "superfoods" with cancer-fighting potential. Each of these possesses its own properties to effectively help with cancer prevention or treatment:

Blueberries
Cinnamon
Grape seed extract
Mushrooms
Pomegranates

Other studies have shown these same foods to have other powerful health-giving properties.

Superfoods help fight other diseases and improve your health. Medical doctors in general practice could recommend these as alternatives or preventive care options for their patients. Afterall, the health of the individual is the goal of medical care, not just the treating of disease.

As is mentioned earlier, frequently grouped under *alternatives* we have two therapies that used to be at the top of the doctor's figurative little black bag - diet and exercise.

The medical profession has long accepted diet and exercise as treatment options for a variety of physical problems. Many doctors, who are not quite so quick to grab the prescription pad, take the time to explain the benefits of these two very natural therapies to their patients.

In the very first medical oath, Hippocrates states, *I will apply dietetic measures for the benefit of the sick according to my ability and judgment; I will keep them from harm and injustice.*

One of the problems of this kind of 'lifestyle' medicine is that it takes time to explain and discuss in order to gain the cooperation of the patient. Face it; it's easier for both the doctor and patient to just agree on a prescription. It may not be healthier, but it is quicker.

However, it is well worth the time it takes to formulate a workable diet and exercise program. By talking with the patient and going over what they eat and drink, the doctor may uncover the source of the complaint. This might take a little more conversation, and won't always work. However, it sure beats unnecessary prescribing or letting the patient run headlong into diabetes or heart disease.

If the physician finds this taking too much time, he or she could recommend a qualified nutritionist. However these are addressed, exercise and proper nutrition are vital tools for disease prevention and as a treatment option for a variety of patient complaints.

The benefits of changes in lifestyle to treat a specific medical problem and increase overall health and wellbeing are numerous. The risks are none. How dangerous could it be to eat well, get enough sleep, and exercise?

Chapter 11
The Alternative of Physical Therapy

Physical therapy is frequently recommended by doctors in hospitals as well as in clinical practice. Physical therapists are highly trained medical specialists. A physical therapist must complete 4 years of college and then get a doctor of physical therapy degree. Many physical therapists also complete a residency program and may also complete a specialty fellowship.

Physical therapy is often considered medically necessary by insurance companies when it is prescribed by an accepted healthcare practitioner. The procedures include therapeutic exercises and joint mobilization. These have generally been shown to be effective in treating aspects of many musculoskeletal conditions.

Physical therapy can be used to treat a wide variety of conditions. If your doctor doesn't mention this form of treatment, ask.

Back and neck problems
Concussion
Headaches
Hip Pain and Arthritis
Jaw pain and dysfunction (TMJ)
Lymphedema
Pain (chronic pain)
Sports Injuries
Urinary Incontinence
Vertigo

Physical therapists provide care for people in a variety of settings, including hospitals, private practices, outpatient clinics, home health agencies, schools, sports and fitness facilities, work settings, and nursing homes.

Whiplash, arthritis, fibromyalgia, degenerative disc disease are other complaints physical therapists are frequently called upon to treat.

PT is routinely an important part of post-operative care and rehab.

The goal of physical therapy is to quickly return the patient to an active life. Physical therapists also work with individuals to prevent the loss of mobility before it occurs by developing fitness and wellness oriented programs.

Chapter 12
Interview with Well-Known Physical Therapist
Dimitrios Kostopoulos, Co-Founder, PT, PhD, DSc, ECS

1. Do patients ever come to see you on recommendation from their medical doctor?

Yes. Some physicians may refer a patient directly to our office and others may provide a list of physical therapy offices for the patients to choose. Many other times a physician may direct the patient to select a therapist based on their insurance directory.

2. What type of problems are you normally called upon to treat?

Musculoskeletal problems such as back and neck pain, arthritis, knee and hip problems, shoulder, elbow and hand problems, sports injuries and others.

3. Can you tell me about a specific time you worked with a patient who had been advised by their doctor to receive physical therapy for a particular complaint, illness, or disease? How was this beneficial to everyone involved?

John, a 38 year old taxi driver, visited my office a few months ago after his medical doctor referred him for physical therapy to take care of his back pain. John presented with lots of pain in the back, radiating to his leg. His symptoms appeared gradually as for the past 3 months he had been working extra long hours to pay for his daughter's college tuition. Sitting and driving a taxi for 15 hrs a day can take a toll on the body. The muscles become tight, they compress on the nerves and pain can become unbearable. A thorough evaluation of his condition and a precise treatment that included manual physical therapy resolved his problem in less than two weeks. Now, John feels fine and he knows what to do to maintain his body in good condition.

4. What would you say is the best part of working with patients who have been sent to you by their doctors?

The fact that we can help patients effectively even with the most difficult problems that others have given up on, provides us with great satisfaction that we have done our duty. And we live for moments like these.

5. What types of health problems have you found success in treating with physical therapy?

Musculoskeletal problems such as back and neck pain, arthritis, knee and hip problems, shoulder, elbow and hand problems, sports injuries and others.

6. How do you feel patients benefit from their doctors explaining the alternative treatments available for their condition?

It is important that they do so. And it is important that physicians have been informed about a variety of alternative treatments and the real evidence as to what alternative treatments work for what conditions.

7. Is there anything else you'd like to tell patients about the importance of Informed Consent and why it matters so much to their health?

It's your body. You have to choose what you want to do about your health, but make sure you only make your decision after you have been given ALL the data.

8. Is there anything you would like to tell doctors regarding explaining to their patients the option of physical therapy to resolve their condition?

Physical therapy is a treatment approach that is absolutely harmless for the patient especially compared to drugs or surgery.

Dimitrios Kostopoulos, Co-Founder, PT, PhD, DSc, ECS

A world renowned, leading expert and best selling author in Myofascial Pain and co-founder of the Hands-On Companies (Est. 1992 in New York). http://www.handsonpt.org

Dr. Kostopoulos has extensive training and teaching experience in different areas of manual therapy with emphasis in Trigger Point, MyoFascial, NeuroFascial Therapy and Manipulation.

He earned his Doctorate (PhD) and Master's degrees at New York University and his second Doctorate of Science (DSc) degree at Rocky Mountain University (Clinical Electrophysiology). Dr. Kostopoulos has obtained his MD degree as a medical graduate from UHSA School of Medicine.

Chapter 13
Naturopathic Medicine as an Alternative to Drugs

Naturopathic physicians generally complete a 4-year, graduate-level program at one of the North American naturopathic medical schools accredited by the Council on Naturopathic Medical Education, an organization recognized for accreditation purposes by the U.S. Department of Education. These doctors are trained to work in hospitals, private practice, clinics, and health centers.

Naturopathic doctors treat most medical conditions and can provide both individual and family health care.

Among the most common ailments they treat are:
Allergies
Chronic Pain
Disgestive Issues
Fatigue
Hormonal Imbalances
Obesity
Respiratory Conditions
Insomnia
Cancer
Heart Disease
Fertility Problems
Menopause
Fibromyalgia

Naturopathic Doctors can perform minor surgeries such as stitching up superficial wounds or removing cysts. They are trained to utilize prescription drugs, although the emphasis of naturopathic medicine is the use of natural healing agents and treatment approaches such as:

Diet Recommendations
Nutritional Supplements
Herbs
Exercise
Counseling
Detoxification
Manipulative Therapies
Homeopathy
Lifestyle Changes
Stress Reduction Techniques

*"Here's good advice for practice:
go into partnership with nature;
she does more than half the work
and asks none of the fee."
- Martine H. Fischer
Physician and Teacher*

Chapter 14
Traditional Chinese Medicine

Traditional Chinese Medicine is an ancient set of practices from China that operate under the belief that the processes of the human body are interrelated and connected to the environment. Practitioners approach healthcare from a holistic standpoint, looking for the underlying imbalances and disharmonies behind an illness.

The practitioner is trained to look at the whole picture and try to treat the patient, instead of just the disease.

Traditional Chinese Medicine originated out of Taoist beliefs established over 4,000 years ago. Today it has been refined and adapted, but many of the practices are performed as they have been for thousands of years.

Traditional Medicine has always been an important component of healthcare in China, and over the past few decades, has grown in popularity in the Western world as well. Today, practices such as acupuncture, T'ai Chi and herbal treatments can be found in many health centers, and scientific studies have shown promising health benefits. Traditional Chinese Medicine has expanded to include diet, nutrition, exercise, spirituality, as well as acupressure.

Chapter 15
Homeopathy as an Alternative Worth Exploring

Homeopathy was one of the most common medical practices in the United States in the 1800s and homeopaths controlled many hospitals, dispensaries, and nursing homes. Now, this form of medical practice is far more prevalent and accepted in Europe than in the U.S. In fact, many countries in Europe are far more open to a variety of health practices. For instance in Germany, the government mandated that all medical school curricula include information about natural medicines. About 10 percent of German doctors specialize in homeopathy, and 10 percent more prescribe homeopathic remedies on occasion. Similar acceptance can be found in the U.K., Switzerland, Italy, Spain, Eastern Europe, France, and Ireland.

Depending on the situation and the practitioner, homeopathic remedies are used by themselves or in conjunction with conventional medicine to treat a wide variety of conditions.

Chapter 16
Ayurvedic Medicine

Ayurvedic medicine, also known as Ayurveda was developed thousands of years ago in India. It's one of the world's oldest whole-body healing systems. In some countries, such as India, Ayurveda is a primary healing system. In the United States it's considered a form of complementary and alternative medicine. Ayurvedic medicine is used primarily to promote good health, rather that to fight disease. Sometimes treatments may be recommended for specific health problems.

Some Ayurvedic Treatments are:

Aromatherapy
Breathing exercises
Diet changes
Herbs
Plant-based oils and spices
Lifestyle changes
Massage
Metals
Minerals
Meditation
Stretching
Vitamins
Yoga

Chapter 17
Mind-body Therapies

Never to be discounted in their ability to heal the body and spirit, mind-body techniques strengthen the communication between the mind and the body. Complementary and Alternative practitioners say these two systems must be in harmony for the individual to stay healthy. Examples of mind-body connection techniques include Tai Chi, meditation, prayer, relaxation techniques, other religions, support of friends and family, Dianetics, and art therapies. Something as simple as taking a walk and looking around at the environment could be considered a mind-body therapy and can significantly improve mood and outlook on life.

Chapter 18
Tai Chi is Another Well-Accepted Alternative

Originally a Chinese martial art, Tai Chi has become a popular mind-body practice. When the person practices Tai Chi, he or she slowly and gently moves their body with awareness of each motion, while engaging in deep breathing. Tai Chi is a low-impact, weight-bearing exercise that improves physical conditioning and balance, eases pain and stiffness, increases mental focus, and enhances overall well being.

The City of Hope and other highly respected American hospitals recommend Tai Chi to their patients who have been weakened by illness or intensive therapy.

Medical researchers have long documented the physical benefits of Tai Chi for those suffering a variety of chronic diseases, including cancer.

A recent study found that tai chi's slow, fluid movements consistently helped middle-aged and older adults improve their walking speed and strength, and in some cases reduced pain and stiffness.

Tai chi oxygenates the tissue and makes breathing more efficient. It improves balance, strength and bone density. It also helps the individual achieve a more peaceful state of mind, which puts them in a much better position to deal with and fight whatever physical and emotional challenges they are facing.

Chapter 19
Yoga is Another Popular Alternative

Another extremely well recognized mind-body therapy is yoga. Yoga is a mental and spiritual practice as well as a physical discipline. This therapy typically involves a combination of physical poses, deep breathing techniques and meditation. Research has indicated that yoga may offer a wide variety of health benefits including relieving stress, reducing pain, and increasing overall health.

Humana, the giant health insurance company, on their website, MyWell-Being.com, has this to say about the benefits of Yoga.

"Dedicating yourself to yoga can be a life-changing experience. The stretching, breathing exercises, relaxation techniques, and mindful meditation involved in this ancient practice offer many potential health benefits for your body and mind."

The same article lists eight benefits to be derived from the practice of yoga.

Yoga can improve your physical fitness and improve balance and posture

Yoga can reduce stress and increase focus and attention

The practice of yoga may improve a person's mental abilities and problem solving abilities

Yoga may be a natural antidepressant, boosting mood and raising spirits

Regular yoga practice can be good for the heart, lowering blood pressure, slowing the heart rate, and improving circulation

Yoga may help relieve chronic pain and increase flexibility

Yoga can help reduce physical tension and relieve insomnia

Yoga may play a role in increasing fertility.

Yoga is a powerful, drug-less form of physical healing that should be something your doctor knows about and can recommend, or at least discuss when it seems appropriate.

Chapter 20
Interview With Noted Author and Yoga Instructor
Kyczy Hawk

1. In your practice are you ever called upon to work with people whose doctors have recommended yoga as part of their overall medical treatment program?

Yes. The yoga I teach is not your garden variety fast paced *vinyasa* (a popular form of yoga frequently taught in yoga classes. It is a slower paced more mindful approach to the poses using body awareness and breath control. This style of yoga is a traditional static poses and flow that is not athletic or challenge based. A conventional gym or studio based yoga class may not provide the same benefits.

2. What type of problems have you been called upon to help?

Active addiction and other mental and emotional disturbances. When you remove the substance you are left with the pre-existing condition. That itself may have been exacerbated by years of intoxication and or disruptive lifestyle choices such as sexual addiction, debt, or gambling.

Stress release, trauma release, conscious breath control as well as enhanced body awareness are only a few of the benefits of a yoga practice.

In time, the body becomes more comfortable AND practiced in alternative stress release methods (deep breathing, stretching, knowing when to rest, recognition of "gut feelings" and so on.)

2a. Can you relate any particular situation that comes to mind where yoga has assisted a person who was dealing with a medical condition?

In addition to addressing the anxiety and physical discomforts that accompany detoxing from chemicals including alcohol, yoga can help those who are experiencing other related issues such as fibromyalgia, chronic fatigue and other immune related diseases and syndromes. Even simple, but painful problems, like plantar fasciitis can be relieved without medication.

3. What was it like working with patients at the Kaiser hospital pain clinic?

As a yoga teacher I was surprised by how intensely restrictive and yet "addictive" chronic pain can be. Without other ways to handle life situations pain itself may become the "way out" of having to face and deal with life. Medications become
both a mask and a lure. They cover the issues, and then become ineffective causing the patient to seek more and higher doses.

Small movements, the tiniest of repeated movements, allowed each person to begin to trust their body again. With regular sessions each person was able to move not necessarily MORE (although that certainly happened) but with less fear
and more enthusiasm. Nutrition and movement such as yoga were very helpful in re-associating the patients with their bodies in a friendlier more integrative way.

3a. How does Yoga work to help people with pain relief?

Some pain is resistance; some is predictive (I hurt last time I did this, so I will avoid that movement and not try it again.). I have a private student I have been working with for a few years. Initially she was very resistive to any sensation -
feeling anything equaled pain, equaled avoidance. Knee pain, plantar fasciitis, wrist and hand pain, hip pain- she presented with them all. She is now working on strength and resistance training as she loses her unwanted weight. She is no
longer living on (over-the-counter) OTC pain medicine and no longer seeks medication from her doctor. She has worked hard at learning to tolerate discomfort and to know what "dangerous" or potentially injurious feelings are. In doing so her life has opened back up to her and she can go to the park and enjoy walks on the beaches again.

4. Can you tell us a little about how the practice of yoga works to help patients in need of mental or emotional relief?

The power of the breath and the information of breath rhythms is very powerful. If we can spot how our breath is changing as we become anxious AND have some practiced methods of controlling the breath, we can calm the mind. Practicing
yoga with full body awareness can give one another predictive tool in sorting out one's feelings and reactions. It takes time - so one or two classes won't get there. I have had students who have dealt with crippling self-esteem issues.

I give a certain cue during poses to bring attention to the mid belly (solar plexus area) which in yoga terms is the third chakra, the seat of self awareness and self esteem. They found that remembering that cue of standing or sitting straight with
support had, over time, given them a sense of empowerment. I had no idea they would experience that so effectively - one for one they related that experience to me.

With self-esteem and an integrated sense of self being at the root of many mental challenges this was great news. It affected how they related to situations in a more positive way.

I have worked with people who have reduced their medications and others who have decided to do without it at all. They did this with their doctor's assistance.

They attribute this desire to the tools they learned in yoga to their desire to make these changes.

5. Do you feel alternative medical practices, including yoga, have been gaining acceptance within the medical community?

I absolutely do. I am in the process of developing an association with a medical group in the San Jose area. I work with other yoga teachers who specialize in yoga for people in cancer treatment, survivors, and their families. Yoga is part of the pain treatment program at our local Kaiser, and we team up with physical therapists to help people recovering from injuries. I have worked with football players from national teams, and other athletes.

While my specialty is addiction recovery the skills are transferable to many areas.

6. Is there anything else you'd like to tell people about the importance of Informed Consent and why it matters so much to their health to be told about alternatives like yoga?

Healthy non-invasive and non- medicative options should always be offered as an adjunct if not an alternative. The younger we can start accepting and believing the messages, the TRUE messages our bodies are telling us, the better off we will be.

When doctors and nurses begin, themselves, to experience the benefits of "alternative" (what I like to call "original" practices, like yoga), the more authentically they can recommend them.

Kyczy Hawk RYT E-500
Author " *Yoga and the Twelve Step Path*" and " *Life in Bite-Sized Morsels*" and " *From Burnout to Balance*" among others.

Kyczy has been teaching recovery focused yoga classes since 2008. Taking the foundation of a traditional yoga training she received from the Lotus Yoga Teacher

Chapter 21
Some Diagnoses Known to Respond Well to Alternative Approaches

The usual treatment for some of the more common medical complaints comes with serious risks. In fact, when patients begin insisting on being told *all* the risks connected with the treatment, they are likely to want to be informed about as many known alternatives as they possibly can. This is where insistence on Informed Consent may prove to be a lifesaver and might eventually make doctors more aware of the risks of current treatments (now that he or she has to say them out loud).

Obviously, some common treatments are just fine. If you have a broken bone, there's no realistic alternative to having it set. If you have a bronchial infection, chances are you're not going to worry about alternatives to the doctor's prescription for antibiotics.

However, for some conditions the usual treatment comes with such serious risks that education in alternative approaches becomes vital.

Two health problems where the dangers and side effects of treatment are huge and which are known to respond well to alternatives are chronic pain and mental health conditions, including a host of psychiatric labels.

Chapter 22
Special Note About Treatments for Pain

Over 100 million U.S. adults suffer from chronic pain.

Pain is a significant problem for many, many people and only the sufferer truly knows how much pain they're in. Sometimes, prescription painkillers are needed on a short-term basis to alleviate this pain. After surgery, for a limited time after an injury, or for intractable cancer pain, prescription pain relievers may offer much needed relief.

However, when a patient comes in complaining of aches and pains, not diagnosed and stemming from an otherwise treatable condition, a physician needs to think in terms of alternatives before writing a prescription. Given enough information, I think most patients would choose to try another option before taking pain pills.

The most frequently recommended treatments for pain are either over-the-counter pain relievers or a prescription.

Pain pills come with very real dangers and prescription pain relievers have been overprescribed and are very addictive, so much so that we currently are fighting an opioid addiction epidemic across the United States.

Millions of people suffering from long-term chronic pain such as lower back pain, arthritis, shoulder and neck pain or nerve pain are prescribed opioid pain relievers, despite there being a surprising lack of medical evidence supporting their successful use in these situations.

Besides not treating long-term pain very well, opioids can cause side effects, including constipation, sedation, overdose, dependence, addiction and death.

Here are some statistics:

Drug overdose is the leading cause of accidental death in the US, with 47,055 lethal drug overdoses in 2014 (the most recent year for which there are statistics).

Overdoses from prescription medications are more frequent than overdoses from street drugs.

Opioid addiction is driving this epidemic, with 18,893 overdose deaths related to prescription pain relievers in 2014.

Painkiller prescription rates are out of control. The total number of opioid pain relievers prescribed in the United States has skyrocketed in the past 25 years The number of prescriptions for opioids (like hydrocodone and oxycodone products) have escalated from around 76 million in 1991 to nearly 207 million in 2013, with the United States their biggest consumer globally.

The point is, pain relief is good, but when that same relief can lead to addiction and death, this is not such a good thing.

Government advice to physicians about prescribing painkillers

Over continuous objections from the pharmaceutical industry and groups that receive their financial support, such as U.S. Pain Foundation and American Academy of Pain Management, Federal and State governments have been trying to set guidelines to reduce and regulate physician prescribing.

In a recent webinar put on by the Center for Disease Control (CDC), the agency revealed the draft of a dozen new guidelines for physicians to follow when prescribing opioids. The first of these guidelines is *"try not to" prescribe*. The preferred option for chronic non-cancer pain is "non-pharmacological" therapy.

Here are some alternatives that can help your doctor follow this advice:

These various recommended alternative and complementary treatments for pain have been compiled from websites and other publications provided by hospitals and insurance companies such as Humana, City of Hope, The Mayo Clinic, and Johns Hopkins. (The resources from which these have been compiled are listed on the website referred to at the end of the book.)

If your doctor does not mention these alternatives, ask him or her about them. It really is part of their job to know enough about them to be able to give you some information relative to the benefits and risks, and recommend a workable alternative or recommend a pain specialist who can.

Alternative Treatments for Pain

Acupuncture

Studies suggest that acupuncture may help with pain relief.

Controlled clinical trials have shown acupuncture to compare favorably with potent, addictive drugs, in the relief of pain. For example:

Acupuncture helps in 55% to 85% of cases
Morphine helps in 70% of cases
Placebo helps in 30% to 35% of cases

Chiropractic to Help With Pain

Research has shown many patients who are suffering from pain can benefit from chiropractic treatment.

Headaches, neck pain, stiff necks, slipped discs, whiplash injuries and even some symptoms connected with fibromyalgia have all been successfully treated with chiropractic manipulation.

Massage

Massage therapy (including Swedish massage, Thai massage, deep tissue massage, and sports massage) relies on touch to treat various parts of your body. Studies suggest that massage helps reduce pain, stress, and tension in the muscles.

Tai Chi

The Chinese practice of Tai Chi involves gentle movements and deep breathing. This low-impact, weight bearing exercise has been found to help ease body pain, headaches, strains, and stiffness and improve physical conditioning and strength.

Tai Chi may also be helpful in relieving anxiety, digestive disorders, soft tissue strains, and headaches. The mental focus involved may also have a significant affect on the perception of pain and discomfort the person experiences.

Physical Therapy

Physical therapists are experts in locating sources of pain and developing treatment plans to address and correct the areas of weakness or stiffness that lie at that source. Physical therapy is aimed at strengthening weakened areas, increasing range of motion and reducing pain. The stronger and more flexible the body becomes, the better its overall alignment, the less pain the person will feel.

Physical therapy or exercise is integral to almost all forms of back and neck pain treatment. Sometimes physical therapists are a first line treatment, other times physical therapists are called upon to help manage chronic pain, or provide rehabilitation after surgery.

Unlike other treatments, such as medication or injections, physical therapy can also help prevent and/or lessen future recurrences of back pain or neck pain.

Yoga

Yoga therapy typically involves a combination of physical poses, deep breathing techniques, and sometimes meditation.

The practice of yoga is known to help reduce or eliminate chronic pain. Yoga can help people with arthritis, fibromyalgia, migraine, low back pain, and many other types of chronic pain conditions.

Considering the side effects, risks and addictive nature that are part of prescription pain relievers, it seems a good idea to give one or more of these alternatives a try before turning to these medications.

Chapter 23
Special Note About Treatments for Emotional, Behavioral, and Mental Health Problems

Another area of patient complaint where alternatives are often sought and thought to be more effective, less risky, and overall healthier than the more frequently recommended treatment is that of mental, behavioral, and emotional health.

The drugs so easily prescribed for these conditions are both powerful and risky. Additionally, it has never been proven that these medications address an actual cause. If you are diagnosed with a psychiatric "disorder" such as anxiety, depression, schizophrenia, bi-polar condition, ask what test was done to establish the medical necessity for a drug. All real medical conditions can be spotted on a blood test, CT scan, or other objective test.

You don't want a drug that simply covers a real medical problem or a treatment that fails to acknowledge there's more to us and to our lives than can or should be suppressed by a pharmaceutical.

If your doctor wants to prescribe a psychoactive drug to you or your child, have him or her explain to you the diagnosis and how it was arrived at, and explain to you in detail the warnings and side effects connected with the drug being prescribed. Also, if the doctor doesn't tell you about alternatives, insist on being told - or find another doctor.

This is from the DePaul Journal of Health Care Law

Informed Consent: Psychiatric Medications, and a Prescribing Physician's Duty to Disclose Safer Alternative Treatments

"The use of psychotropic medication to treat any presumed mental health disorder always involves serious risk of harm. Accordingly, before prescribing psychotropic medication to control the behaviors associated with presumed mental disorder, under various ethical guidelines and Informed Consent laws, prescribing physicians must first disclose available information regarding not only the risks of taking the recommended medication, but also the availability of alternative treatment options, and the risks and benefits of choosing such alternative treatment options. Indeed, given the highly intrusive nature of psychotropic medication and the conceded unknown etiology (causation) of most mental health disorders, disclosing information in support of safer alternative treatments seems a particularly critical aspect of a prescribing physician's Informed Consent obligations in the mental health arena."

<u>Alternative and Complementary Approaches to Mental Health Are Many</u>

<u>Friendship / Religion / Counseling</u>

In the past, when someone was going through a tough time and felt depressed, stressed, worried, sad, anxious, angry, or any of the other multitude of emotions that can bother us as humans, they turned to religion, friendship, or counseling. Drugs would never have been considered as a first line treatment.

And until fairly recently no one would ever have dreamt of giving a child a psychoactive drug in order to alter their behavior. Good control by parents and teachers, counseling, personal attention, proper diet and nutrition, and exercise, would be the courses of "treatment" given to a child.

A Real Medical Problem or Drug Side Effect?

Many illnesses and diseases produce in the individual a feeling of anxiety or depression. When a patient comes into a doctors office seeking help for these types of problems, the first step should be to give them a thorough, physical exam.

I had a friend who was seeking counseling because she felt so down all the time. Luckily, the counselor could see my friend wasn't looking that well physically, and had her go get a physical. It was discovered she had very early stage cancer. She received proper treatment, the cancer was cured, and she no longer felt anxious or depressed. By being alert and perceptive that counselor saved my friend's life.

Many prescription medications have side effects that produce negative effects on the mental and emotional state of the patient. This should be among the first things you and your doctor look into if you are feeling emotionally battered.

Meditation

As I was taking a little break from writing just now, I ran across yet another article about the positive effects meditation has on depression, anxiety and other mental and emotional ills. In the article the author discussed a research study comparing antidepressants to meditation for the relief of depression. The study found that meditation reduced symptoms of stress and depression, and increased in the patients a general sense of well-being - with no side effects.

Major medical centers are offering meditation classes to help people who are suffering with depression or anxiety stemming from treatments such as chemotherapy and radiation.

The point is, meditation is a solution worth looking into before opting to take drugs.

Lifestyle Changes (Diet, Nutrition, and Exercise)

When you see your doctor about emotional or behavioral troubles, make sure you get the opportunity to really talk about what's going on with your life.

How nutritious are the foods you eat? Do you drink too much coffee, sugary beverages, or alcohol? Do you get enough exercise? Do you take walks or get out in the fresh air and sunlight? Do you sleep well?

If your physician doesn't have the time to go over these questions with you, get that doctor to recommend a naturopath or nutritionist.

Study after study has shown the power of these alternatives to treat depression, anxiety, and many forms of stress. And the good news is, these therapies have no negative side effects.

Several other alternatives are available to treat problems with your mood.

Alternative and Complementary Treatments for Depression, Anxiety, Stress, Attention Problems and Other Emotional and Mood Related Difficulties

* Acupuncture
* Counseling
* Dianetics
* Diet and Nutrition
* Exercise
* Herbs
* Homeopathy
* Meditation
* Supplements
* Tai Chi

Dozens of books have been written citing study after study that prove the safety and efficacy of alternatives to prescription medications in treating mood, emotional, and behavioral problems. If your doctor doesn't recommend trying one before putting you on a medication, insist on your right to Informed Consent and being told of alternatives. The information is readily available to your doctor and has widespread agreement from various accepted authorities.

The conditions discussed above are not the only ones that respond well to alternative and complementary medicine.

Chapter 24
Summary of Alternative Treatments Step of Informed Consent

The point of this section on alternatives is not so much the specific treatments and their potential for success, but that there are many, many solutions available to doctors and their patients that must be explored.

Doctors should not think that these "alternatives" are somehow beneath them or out of the realm of western medicine. Well established, recognized medical centers such as City of Hope, the Mayo Clinic, and Johns Hopkins, just to name a few, use many of these complementary and alternative remedies to help their patients. These are conservative hospitals and research centers.

Doctors working at this level would not embrace an alternative treatment if they did not think it would benefit their patients. A medical doctor in clinical practice would be arrogant indeed to think they did not need to investigate and recommend alternative treatments.

Prescribing a drug is easy and quick. There's no need to think outside the box or to spend the time learning something new. Pharmaceutical medications are advertised in all the medical journals and backed up by studies (sometimes paid for by the drug companies). Alternatives require more personal effort and thought.

Given sufficient information, you should have a good idea whether the treatment being offered really makes sense for you. Even if it does, find out about your alternatives anyway. You may want to try one first since no drugs come without substantial risks.

Make sure you insist your doctor tell you about alternatives; if he or she is not aware of any, you may have to educate your physician or find another.

What has been lost over time is the cooperation amongst medical disciplines. Because of this, physicians lost the chance to work with practitioners in other healing arts. The ultimate loser is, of course, the patient.

Doctors should embrace the possibilities for disease prevention and cure these alternatives offer. Working together, all the members of the healing arts will be able to help patients live longer, healthier, and happier lives.

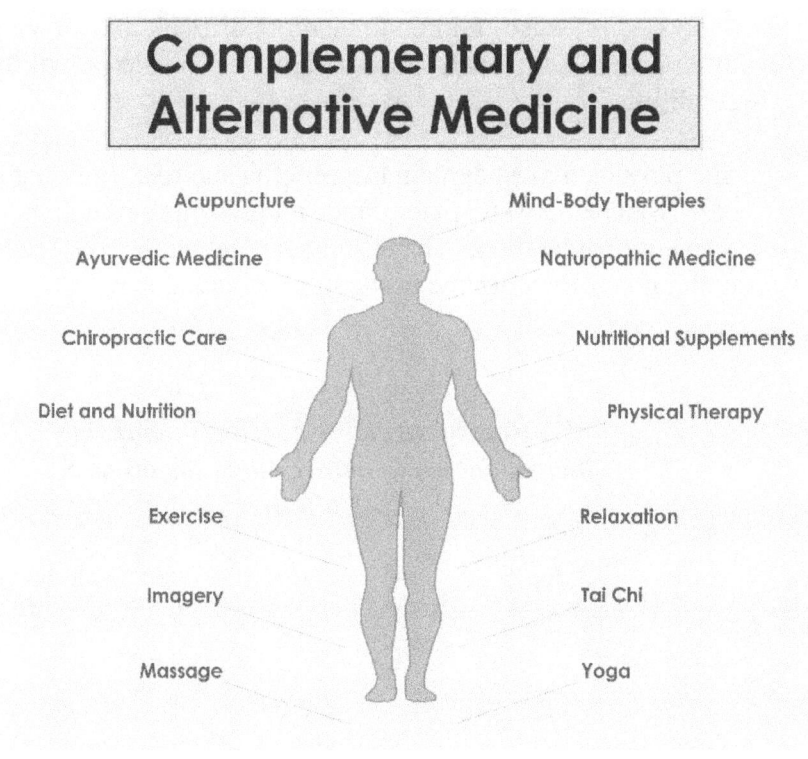

Alternative and Complementary Treatments
Accepted By Major Medical Authorities in U.S. and Abroad

Chapter 25
What Happens if I Do Nothing?

As part of Informed Consent, your doctor must tell you about the risks and benefits of doing nothing.

Many conditions do cure themselves. Sometimes a cold or flu just needs to run its course and, with bed rest and fluids, will be gone in a few days to a couple of weeks.

And sometimes the stresses of life cause us to feel anxious or depressed or cause children to be more difficult to handle. More often than not, time and simple solutions can take care of these conditions.

The physician must explain the benefits and risks of doing nothing or a "watch and wait" plan. Since all prescriptions and most other conventional treatments have serious potential side effects, doing nothing is sometimes the best course of action.

"The art of medicine consists in amusing the patient while nature cures the disease."
- Voltaire

Chapter 26
How Much Information is Enough?

It's up to the physician to give the patient enough data to make a truly informed decision. But how much information is enough?

Two different standards for the responsible application of Informed Consent are the *reasonable doctor* standard and the *reasonable patient* standard.

The basic principle is that physicians are required to advise their patients of material risks. The definition of a material risk is a risk or adverse effect that is important to the patient; information that would affect the decision-making process of a reasonable person.

Risks that may be trivial but are common and risks that may be rare but are severe must be disclosed. A risk that is severe but rare such as the risk of death and must be disclosed.

You have a right to demand of your doctor that he or she follow the rules of Informed Consent. But certain questions can come up regarding what exactly is being sought and how much information is considered enough to fulfill ethical and legal requirements.

The Reasonable Patient Standard

This standard asserts the Informed Consent communication process should be from the patient's perspective, since it is the patient who is asked to give their consent.

It requires physicians and other health care practitioners to disclose all relevant information about the risks, benefits, and alternatives of a proposed treatment that an average patient would feel they need in order to make an intelligent decision about whether to agree to the proposed procedure or treatment option.

Currently, most Informed Consent discussions fail to offer details about the material risks, and the alternatives that are a critical and meaningful part of the patient's decision-making process.

Without sufficient information, a patient cannot be expected to make an intelligent decision or be a real partner in his or her own care.

The Reasonable Doctor Standard

The reasonable doctor standard holds that a physician need only give the patient the same amount of information that any other doctor would. With this interpretation, doctors are likely to stick up for others doctors, even when the amount of information would be insufficient for any normal patient to feel informed enough to give consent.

Even though this is not a real patient-oriented, high level of caring, type standard, it does not eliminate the need for Informed Consent and still requires that the health practitioner *talk* to the patient and communicate all the required steps. Just because physicians in some parts of the country are held to a lower legal standard of consent, does not eliminate the law, nor the ethical standards connected with a patient's right to determine what is done to his or her body.

An Example

This court case from the UK will show a real life example of the differences between these two standards.

The case was Montgomery v Lanarkshire Health Board heard by the U.K. Supreme Court in 2015.

In this case, a woman with insulin-dependent diabetes, claimed that her obstetrician failed to communicate the risk of shoulder dystocia (a problem with delivery that occurs when the baby has trouble being removed from the mother through her vagina) during vaginal delivery that ultimately resulted in severe fetal brain anoxia (insufficient oxygen to the brain, causing brain damage).

The woman claimed that had she received full information about the risks, she would have decided upon a cesarean delivery. Yet the treating obstetrician (and other expert physicians called to trial) claimed that the ensuing risk was very small and thus appropriately not communicated because a cesarean delivery is not in the maternal interest. The obstetrician reported that "…had I raised it [the risks of shoulder dystocia] with her then yes, she would have no doubt requested a caesarean section, as would any diabetic today."

Finding in favor of the patient, in its final decision, the UK Supreme Court ruled that the standard for what *physicians should inform patients about the risks, benefits, and alternatives of treatment will no longer be determined by what a responsible body of physicians deems important, but rather by what a reasonable patient deems important.*

It would seem to me that, rather than limiting the amount of information that passes between doctor and patient, it would be more appropriate for doctors to learn how to communicate and explain risks, without downplaying the dangers. When a doctor has familiarized himself or herself about alternative treatments, he or she will likely be more willing to discuss the risks of the original treatment recommendation.

It's pretty obvious that most patients are not doctors. A patient cannot be expected to have the education, knowledge or experience of the physician and knowledge of adverse effects or risks cannot be expected. If anything, a doctor should err on the side of too much explaining.

Some doctors express concern that if they give the patient too much information he or she may be afraid of the treatment. In some cases, the patient may be right to be afraid. But it is the patient's decision, not the doctors. Every person has a right to understand and consent to what's going to happen to his or her body. This holds true whether it's the effect of a medication or of a diagnostic procedure, chemotherapy, radiation, surgery, or other medical practice. And the patient deserves to have all the "meaningful" information and to know the truth.

Both the reasonable physician standard and the reasonable patient standard allow for patients requesting more information, a second opinion, or support from a family member or friend in the decision-making process.

Chapter 27
You May Need to Get a Second Opinion

Sometimes doctors get it wrong. The error may be with the diagnosis, with the treatment recommendation, or with their ability to honestly tell patients about benefits, risks, or alternative treatments. Whatever the situation, if you have any doubts, you should get a second opinion.

Even excellent doctors and well-known hospitals can make errors, and far too frequently they do.

Most doctors have no objection to your seeing another physician. It helps them be sure they've gotten it right and if they have, it backs up their decision.

The situation doesn't have to be extreme to warrant a second opinion. Just being told to take a prescription that has more risks than you're comfortable with is reason enough. Or if your doctor is unwilling to discuss alternative or complementary therapies, or simply is unaware of any, might be an indication that a second opinion would be a good idea.

And never be afraid you will hurt your doctor's feelings. Getting a second opinion is part of medical practice. If your doctor had it wrong, he or she will be glad to be corrected.

When to get a second opinion:

* Your doctor does not seem to listen to you.

* Your diagnosis does not make sense to you or is not based on scientific tests, but is more a matter or opinion.

* The suggested treatment is risky and you'd like to see if there's a safer, less drastic solution.

* The doctor seems reluctant to give you all the information you need, but simply expects you to "do as you're told." (This is a violation of the Informed Consent law)

* Your doctor is unable to explain your diagnosis, treatment recommendation, or alternatives to you in a manner you can understand and that will lead to your making an *informed* decision.

* You would feel better getting a second opinion.

Getting a second opinion is the right of any patient and it's better to err on the side of caution than to be shy or embarrassed about seeing another doctor. If he or she is one of the thousands of great well-intentioned doctors who work hard for us in cities and towns across America, they will have no problem with your doing so.

Chapter 28
Exceptions to the Law of Informed Consent

Emergency Exception

The emergency exception is just that--an exception limited to emergencies. These may be in the emergency room, or may involve patients in the hospital who have an unexpected event such as a cardiac arrest.

This exception is based on the premise that any reasonable person would not want to be denied necessary medical care. This applies when the patient is unable to consent, such as when someone is brought unconscious or delirious into an emergency room, and the treatment is needed to save his or her life or prevent permanent disability.

Frequently, this emergency exception involves the treatment of children who are legally unable to consent due to their age. An example of this would be a 12 year old who has broken an arm and is brought to the hospital by a neighbor. Neither the child nor the neighbor is legally able to consent to treatment. The physician may rely on the emergency exception to consent if immediate care is necessary to preserve the use of the child's arm.

A rare abuse of the emergency exception involves patients who have refused to consent to specific medical care. The refusal may be based on religious beliefs, such as refusing blood transfusions, or on a personal decision, such as refusing intensive care. If the physician disagrees with such a decision, the time to fight the decision is when it is made. There is no legal justification for waiting until the patient is unconscious or for physically or chemically restraining a patient and then rendering care against the patient's consent. This would not constitute an emergency exception to the need for consent. On the contrary, it would constitute battery. Obviously, no well-intentioned doctor would engage in this kind of behavior.

Chronically incompetent patients or those patients who are simple less able to understand what is going on with their medical care and treatments should always have a legal guardian. This need has come into prominence lately due to the over-drugging and mistreatment of seniors in some long-term care facilities.

"Psychologically Fragile" Patients

This possible exception to Informed Consent is usually turned down as a defense by the courts. The concept the defense tries to put forth is that if the patient knew the risks of treatment, they wouldn't agree it being done to them. (That's the whole point of Informed Consent. The patient has a right to determine what's going to happen to his or her own body!)

In cases involving mental patients, courts have refused to accept the withholding of information about risks based on concerns that the patients would otherwise refuse the necessary treatments. In one case involving a patient under psychiatric care, the court held that it was improper not to tell the patient about the risk of tardive dyskinesia the treatment could cause.

The defendant physician argued that had the patient been told of the risk, he would have refused the treatment. The court rejected this argument, finding that the policy behind Informed Consent was precisely to allow patients to choose to refuse treatment. If the physician believes that a patient must be deceived into necessary therapy, perhaps the practitioner should find a better treatment.

One of the reasons courts have a narrow interpretation of this "therapeutic" exception is the belief that if a patient is sufficiently psychologically fragile as to be harmed by the consent process, then perhaps that patient is not competent to consent to care and needs a legal guardian to guide them in their choice. This guardianship should not be used just to bypass a patient's right to Informed Consent.

If you are in an emotionally stressful medical situation, have a guardian or advocate available to make sure no one deprives you of your right to Informed Consent. If you have a relative who may not be able to fully understand their medical treatment or care, make sure they have someone to advise and guide them. This will help keep them out of the over-drugging that has become so much a part of the "care" of seniors and other physically or emotionally fragile patients.

The Good Samaritan

Good Samaritan laws were written to cover a special type of situation. Years ago, many doctors coming across the scene of an accident were afraid to stop and help. Frequently not having all their medical equipment with them, these physicians could only do their best with what they had available to handle the medical situation confronting them. Unscrupulous people, taking advantage of this desire on the part of the doctors to help, would later sue for substandard care.

Today, most states have Good Samaritan laws that protect a doctor who stops to help an injured person. In some states a doctor is actually required to stop and offer assistance. So, no matter how bad the results, you cannot sue for Good Samaritan treatment unless you can show the doctor was grossly negligent.

Barriers to Informed Consent

In children's books and TV shows doctors are normally shown to be knowing, patient, wise, and kind; with nothing but our best interests at heart - 'doctor knows best'. As we grow up physicians are still shown in advertising to be the ones who know. "Ask your doctor about…" or "Ask your doctor if____ is right for you" are two recommendations that appear toward the end of almost every pharmaceutical advertisement.

Most doctors are knowledgeable and do care. But doctors are as human as anyone else and studies have shown that they can be swayed and their medical judgment influenced by any number of external pressures and even some temptations.

People need to know their doctors are on the patient's side, not on the side of some known or unknown influence being brought to bear on the physician or the practice of medicine.

The next chapters cover many of the barriers patients and physicians face in ensuring the law of Informed Consent is upheld

Chapter 29
Barrier: Fraudulent Practices and Physician Error

I'd love to believe that government regulatory agencies such as the Food and Drug Administration (FDA) protect us from bad drugs and faulty medical devices. I'd love to think companies that make medical products such as prescription medications and hip replacement devices act for the greater good rather than simple profits and that they're honest in their reporting of clinical trial results and dangerous side effects.

I'd also be truly happy if I knew that no physician ever let their ties to various manufacturing firms guide them in their diagnosis and treatment of patients.

Unfortunately, none of these is true.

Many prescription drugs are both safe and effective, but not all. Most of the devices placed in our bodies do not cause bad reactions, but some do.

When companies hide information about dangerous side effects, lawsuits frequently follow.

Here are some cases where, either through greed or misinformation, patients were given medications or implanted with devices that were unsafe and are now the subject of lawsuits.

Abilify and Complusive Behavior

Despite its known side effects, Abilify (aripirazole) is been prescribed to nearly a million Americans each year. One of the potential side effects, compulsive behavior, has been hidden from patients. People taking this drug have found they are unable to stop themselves from pathological gambling, hypersexual activity, or binge eating, when these were never problems for them before.

For example, people without any previous desire to gamble can find themselves running up their credit cards or mortgaging their homes in order to fulfill this desire. Patients can be so consumed by this behavior that they cannot stop without professional counseling.

While this type of side effect causes no immediate physical harm, it can do untold damage to a person's self respect and to their life.

A growing number of Abilify lawsuits allege that Bristol-Myers Squibb and Otsuka failed to provide patients and doctors with adequate warnings about the risk of compulsive behavior.

Avandia and Heart Attacks

GlaxoSmithKline paid $3 billion in 2012 to settle charges brought by the US Department of Justice concerning its diabetes drug Avandia. The manufacturer had previously paid out at least $750 million in more than 50,000 individual lawsuits and has earmarked $6 billion for future lawsuits related to the drug.

Research demonstrated that Avandia's clinical trials showed an increase risk for heart attacks. The pharmaceutical manufacturer failed to report these results to authorities, hiding them from the doctors who prescribed and the patients who trusted those doctors.

Also in 2012, GlaxoSmithKline pleaded guilty to misbranding two of their antidepressant medications – Wellbutrin and Paxil.

Seroquel Promoted for Unapproved Uses and Seroquel and Diabetes

The drug maker AstraZeneca paid a $68.5 million settlement in 2011 over complaints their anti-psychotic medication Seroquel was promoted for unapproved uses. The settlement related to cases in nearly 40 states and the District of Columbia.

Claims have also been made regarding Seroquel as causing diabetes. AstraZeneca has earmarked nearly $650 million to resolve lawsuits related to these claims.

Zyprexa Promoted for Unapproved Uses and Failing to Communicate Severity of Side Effects

Zyprexa (olanzapine) is an antipsychotic drug made by Eli Lilly & Co. It has been prescribed to over 20 million people since it was approved by the FDA in 1996.

Over 18,000 lawsuits have been filed by people who were injured by Zyprexa. Eli Lilly marketed their drug for unapproved uses, including prescribing it to children and for older people with dementia, and downplaying the risk of side effects.

In 2007, Eli Lilly agreed to pay $500 million to resolve the litigation. In total, the company paid $1.2 billion to 28,500 people who experienced severe side effects.

Two years later, the company paid $1.42 billion to settle civil and criminal investigations into illegal "off-label" marketing with the Justice Department and several states.

The drug company made hundreds of millions of dollars by convincing doctors to prescribe Zyprexa in unapproved dosages and for unapproved uses, putting thousands upon thousands of patients at risk.

Lipitor and Diabetes

Millions of people have been prescribed Lipitor with the expectation of controlling cholesterol. (Whether or not this prescribing is necessary is a frequent subject of debate amongst health care providers.) However, what's not under debate is that patients prescribed Lipitor did not expect to develop Diabetes.

However, according to a 2012 warning by the U.S. Food and Drug Administration (FDA), some cholesterol-reducing statins, including Lipitor, may increase the risks of elevated blood sugar levels and developing type-2 diabetes. The FDA ordered Pfizer, the maker of Lipitor, to add warnings about diabetes risks to Lipitor's labels.

This warning came too late for many people who suffered serious side effects from taking Lipitor. Many have filed lawsuits against Pfizer because of their injuries. More lawsuits are expected.

Kickbacks for Diabetic Management Products

Prescription drugs are not the only medical treatment capable of putting consumers at risk and triggering legal settlements. A number of companies face lawsuits based on their medical devices. These devices include surgical implants, prosthetics, and tools intended to stabilize health issues.

In 2008, the Bayer corporation paid nearly $100 million to settle allegations the company had paid kickbacks to its suppliers of diabetic management products. The lawsuit alleged Bayer engaged in a cash-for-patient scheme that bribed suppliers to choose Bayer products over other options.

Patients are usually not trained in the medical field and must rely on the advice of their doctors and the marketing claims made by companies they believe are selling safe products.

Patients are responsible for their own health, but naturally most people put a great deal of weight on the recommendation of their doctor when making a choice of treatments. Unfortunately, when companies market their products to doctors and form an unethical relationship between a medical device company or prescription drug manufacturer and a physician, it's the patients that pay the price.

Chapter 30
Industry Lobbying in Washington

One of the barriers to the correct application of Informed Consent comes from the power of money to influence those who serve us in Washington.

The *Center for Responsive Politics* (Opensecrets.org) keeps track of money paid by lobbyists representing various sectors of industry to our congressmen and congresswomen in order to influence our government and protect their own interests.

Here's a chart taken (with permission) from Center for Responsive Politics. I think it tells the story. It may explain why the health products industry is so out of control.

Lobbying - Top Industries 2015

Pharmaceuticals/Health Products	$231,318,911
Insurance	$157,221,882
Oil & Gas	$129,836,004
Business Associations	$129,098,164
Electronics Mfg & Equip	$122,158,480
Electric Utilities	$117,715,016
Misc Manufacturing & Distributing	$104,937,266
Securities & Investment	$97,848,863
Hospitals/Nursing Homes	$92,993,765
Telecom Services	$90,801,758
Health Professionals	$89,841,202
Air Transport	$81,482,628
Real Estate	$77,811,327
Education	$77,102,754
Defense Aerospace	$74,446,775
Health Services/HMOs	$73,236,898
Civil Servants/Public Officials	$71,155,628
Commercial Banks	$64,872,735
TV/Movies/Music	$62,142,091
Automotive	$58,759,623

Source: Center for Responsive Politics, www.opensecrets.org based on documents obtained from the Federal Election Commission

Chapter 31
Astroturfing as a Marketing Plan

Part of the crazy marketing and lobbying genius of pharmaceutical manufacturing firms, involves the use of fraudulent front groups to help them gain credibility for their "diseases" and cooperation from government.

The use of these front groups has been termed "astroturfing"; an expression used to refer to a fake grass roots movement. Astroturfing involves an organization masquerading as a grass roots movement while hiding the true sponsor, intentions, and motives behind this curtain. These fake groups and movements seek to sway public opinion and governmental oversight by promoting "causes" that benefit the corporation behind the curtain.

New front groups are constantly being created and used to mold public opinion and lobby for support. These groups create the illusion of generalized need and support for their product or general antagonism to anything seeking to weaken their power.

Here is a list of just some of those front groups. Many of these are or have been under investigation by the Senate for their huge amounts of previously undisclosed pharmaceutical funding.

American Foundation for Suicide Prevention
Anxiety Disorders Association of America (ADAA)
Attention Deficit Disorder Association (ADDA)
Center for the Advancement of Children's Mental Health (CACMH)
Children and Adults with ADD (CHADD)
Depression and Bipolar Support Alliance (DBSA)
DBSA Advisory Board
Mental Health America (Formerly National Mental Health Association)
National Alliance on Mental Illness (NAMI)
National Association for Research on Schizophrenia And Depression (NARSAD)

Screening for Mental Health, Inc

Signs of Suicide (SOS)
Suicide Prevention Action Network USA (SPAN)
TeenScreen National Center for Mental Health Checkups
The Jed Foundation

One of the groups under investigation is the *National Alliance on Mental Illness*, one of America's most influential disease advocacy groups. Congressional investigators discovered that a majority of the donations made to the *National Alliance on Mental Illness* (NAMI) have come from drug makers in recent years.

While pretending to be an advocacy group, lobbying efforts of the *National Alliance on Mental Illness* are aimed at pushing legislation that benefits the drug manufacturing industry.

Meanwhile, investigation continues into other influential disease and patient advocacy groups and organizations with regards to their ties to drug and device manufacturers; all part of the investigation into the drug industry's influence on the practice of medicine.

Chapter 32
Pharmaceutical Advertising to Doctors

One of the largest barriers to our receiving the best possible medical care lies in the sway pharmaceutical manufacturers hold over physicians.

The influence of pharmaceutical companies over doctors begins in school and continues all the way through to retirement. If you ask any doctor whether their prescribing patterns can be changed by a free lunch or a bottle of wine, he or she would say, certainly not. However, research shows otherwise.

Medical schools offer one of the first avenues of contact between students and pharmaceutical companies. Maybe it's not so surprising, that the more contact doctors have with pharmaceutical companies and their representatives, the more likely they are to think it doesn't affect prescribing behavior.

In a study done of medical residents, more than half felt they were immune to drug company promotions, but only 16% felt other physicians could remain uninfluenced by these same promotions. This means those residents felt that while they are not affected by pharma marketing, other doctors are.

Payments, in one form or another, to physicians across the United States, have for many years been out of hand. Nearly 9 in 10 cardiologists who wrote at least 1,000 prescriptions for Medicare patients received payments from a drug or medical device company in 2014, while 7 in 10 internists and family practitioners did as well.

For some reason, despite all the evidence to the contrary, doctors continue to insist the lunches, "consulting" fees, and other gifts from the pharmaceutical industry have no effect on their prescribing habits. Does a hypnotized man know he's been hypnotized? Does the victim of a con know they've been conned?

The pharmaceutical industry has been a friendly part of these doctors' lives for far too long.

Look at the brochures, placed in a rack in your doctor's office. These will tell you about a disease, "disorder", or illness. Then, usually after a short, vague section about diet and exercise, these brochures tout the marvels of some brand-name prescription medication. And who gives these wonderful pamphlets to the doctor? Look for the fine print; every one of these is given out by the very drug company that sells that drug.

Well-dressed, attractive, drug company reps with bright smiles, haunt the halls of medical buildings, doctor's waiting rooms, and hospitals in hopes of persuading doctors to write more prescriptions for their company's (expensive) brand name drugs. In far too many cases those hopes are easily fulfilled. A free lunch is enough to do the trick.

Doctors attend conferences and lectures with lunches paid for by the pharmaceutical industry.

Written information and pharma-sponsored events provided by drug companies are a staple of continuing education for doctors. Journal advertisements by drug companies and pharmaceutical company sponsored clinical trials make their way into a doctor's frame of reference when he or she is looking for a solution to a patient's problem. And all lead to an increase in the prescribing of the promoted drug.

Research studies are published where the investigators have received grants from drug companies. Positive results are widely published; unfavorable ones somehow don't see the light of day.

Pens, "informative" materials, notepads, clocks, and coffee mugs, sporting names like Lipitor, Seroquel, Merck, and Pfizer are ubiquitous in medical facilities.

Free drug samples of the latest brand-name product or any other drug currently slated for promotion line the cupboards of most doctors' offices.

If all this marketing didn't work, pharmaceutical companies wouldn't do it.

Ad spending by drug manufacturers soared more than 60 percent in the last four years, hitting $5.2 billion last year (2014). (This doesn't include drug reps, free samples, journal articles, and all the other forms of pharmaceutical marketing.)

Even with all the money drug manufacturers spend telling consumers to, "ask your doctor about….", most of the marketing money is directed at the physicians that do the prescribing.

Drug companies spent more than $3 billion a year marketing to consumers in the U.S. in 2012, and an estimated $24 billion marketing directly to health care professionals.

Drug companies also spend far more on marketing than they do on research. According to an article in the Huffington Post, May 8, 2013, pharmaceutical companies spend 19 times more on promotion than on basic research.

Pharmaceutical companies are, after all, at their core, businesses. These businesses want to make all the profits they can.

Even the American Medical Association is getting tired of the influence that Big Pharma advertising has on the American public. In 2015 the AMA called for a ban on direct-to-consumer advertising by drug companies. This association has yet to realize how their own doctors are affected by the same kind of persuasion created by constant marketing, but at least this is a start.

After being barraged since the beginning of their medical education by clever and persistent pharmaceutical marketing, it's no wonder physicians prescribe so many medications and turn a deaf ear to alternative approaches. But, the health of their patients and the effectiveness of our healthcare system depend on unbiased health advice. It's hard to imagine this happening as long as the tendrils of big pharma reach to deep into every part of our medical care.

It doesn't matter whether or not doctors recognize that their prescribing behavior is influenced by the constant onslaught of marketing from the pharmaceutical industry, it is the patient that suffers by receiving biased advice. And it is the patient, as well as the broader health care system that pays for unnecessarily expensive newer drugs when often less expensive generic alternatives or no drugs at all, would work just as well.

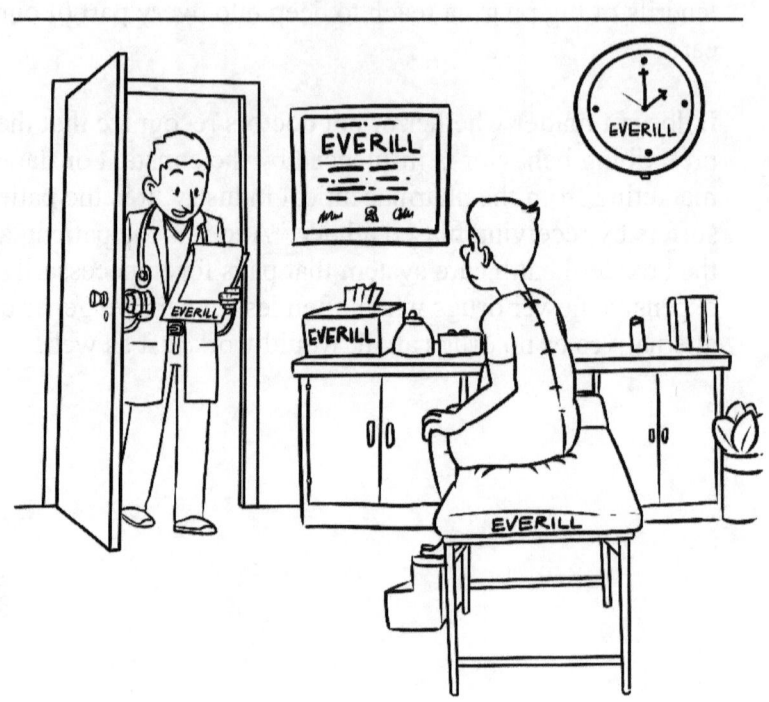

I have just the drug for you ... Everill.

Chapter 33
Conflicts of Interest

A conflict of interest arises when a person's personal interests conflict with their professional duties. This conflict can make their decisions unreliable. The conflicting interest could be money, status, reputation, or anything else desirable to the individual.

In the case of medicine, the primary interest must always be the patient. In a conflict of interest the risk is that what is best for the patient may be relegated to second place over the interests of a pharmaceutical firm, device manufacturer or other healthcare product or service provider.

One concern regarding the practice of medicine is to protect the judgment of the individual physician from undue influence. Whether the risk arises from kickbacks, gifts, personal relationships, personal gain (either financial or in status or recognition), or the interests of family, colleagues, or current or former patients, most doctors have no idea they are even being influenced.

> *"A physician shall not receive any financial benefits or other incentives solely for referring patients or prescribing specific products."*
> *- World Medical Association*
> *International Code of Medical Ethics*

Unfortunately, doctors can develop relationships with pharmaceutical and medical device companies or their representatives. Some doctors are even part owners in medically related firms.

Doctors can make extra money by becoming promotional speakers or writers on behalf of drug manufacturers. They may have a financial interest in a medical company whose product they prescribe, use, or recommend.

Whether the physician is aware of it or not, the gifts and financial compensation given to them by drug companies and their representatives do have an effect on their treatment choices. These relationships cannot help but create a conflict of interest in the physician.

Even when the gift from a drug company representative is as small as a dozen pens or a $20 lunch, it's a natural human impulse, to want to give something back to the giver.

Find out if your doctor has any financial ties to the company that makes the medication he or she is prescribing; this could be anything from a few free lunches to tens of thousands in "consulting" or speaking fees.

Take a look around the office. Are there any pamphlets, papers, or objects with the name of a drug company or medication printed on them? Is your doctor writing the prescription with a pen that has a pharmaceutical company slogan emblazoned on it?

These are all indicators of a drug rep infiltrated office and may mean the doctor relies heavily on the salespeople and flashy brochures for information regarding new drugs, rather than careful review of the scientific data.

Until such time as our doctors have no financial ties of any kind to the companies that make the products they recommend, we must protect the integrity of medicine by getting the disclosure of doctor's financial relationships with these companies. Once these ties are revealed, the patient can then use the information to decide if they want to agree to the proposed treatment or get another opinion from a physician who does not have these ties.

In a report entitled "Conflict of Interest in Medical Research, Education, and Practice" from the National Academy of Sciences the committee called upon physicians to "directly adopt practices that are consistent with high levels of professionalism".

These recommendations include (taken verbatim from the report):

* not accept items of material value from pharmaceutical, medical device, and biotechnology companies except when a transaction involves payment at fair market value for a legitimate service;

* not make educational presentations or publish scientific articles that are controlled by industry or contain substantial portions written by someone who is not identified as the author or who is not properly acknowledged;

* not enter into consulting arrangements unless they are based on written contracts for expert services to be paid for at fair market value;

* not meet with pharmaceutical and medical device sales representatives except by documented appointments and at the physician's express invitation;

* not accept drug samples except in specified situations for patients who lack financial access to medications.

Health care providers should establish policies for their employees and medical staff that are consistent with these recommendations. - from National Academies Press Report ISBN 978-0-309-13188-9

Any questions or conflicts between the interest of the patient and other interests should always be resolved by the physician in favor of the patient.

Chapter 34
Drugs You Don't Need for Diseases You Don't Have
Pharmaceutical Advertising to Consumers

In the United States drug advertising has become part of our cultural tapestry. Just because this advertising has become so normal to us, doesn't mean it is a normal (or responsible) way of informing the public about diseases and medical options. In fact, the U.S. and New Zealand are the only two developed countries in the world that allow drug companies to advertise directly to consumers. Unfortunately, this aggressive advertising works. Citizens of these two countries take more prescription medications than those of any other country.

This advertising puts more stress on doctors, because patients come in having already been convinced that one little pill will "cure" them of just about anything.

In a, now famous study, researchers in Canada and United States looked at the effects of direct-to-consumer advertising on patients in two demographically similar cities; Vancouver and Sacramento. They discovered that U.S. consumers, constantly hit by prescription drug advertising, were twice as likely to ask their doctors for a drug they heard about than were the consumers in Canada, where such advertising is not allowed.

This advertising affects all aspects of our care.

In a 2014 study, reported in *Science Daily*, actors, playing the part of patients, visited physicians complaining of either sciatica or knee arthritis. Half the "patients" with sciatica specifically requested the powerful narcotic painkiller, oxycodone. Half the "patients" with knee arthritis requested the prescription drug Celebrex. The other half of the "patients" in each group requested, "just something to make it better."

About 20% of the sciatica "patients" requesting oxycodone received it, compared to 1 percent of those making no such specific request. As a note, strong narcotic pain killers, such as Oxycodone are generally not recommended for sciatica, especially a new case, such as these were.

About half of knee arthritis patients requesting Celebrex receive that drug, compared to one-fourth of those requesting no specific medication.

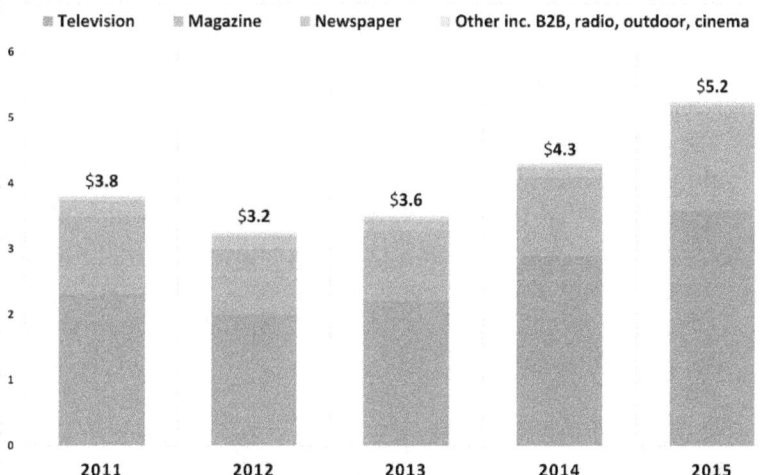

Figures in Billions
Digital Outlets Not Included
Source: Nielsen

Since direct to consumer advertising became legal in 1985 the prescribing rate for the advertised drug has risen to 34.2% while non-advertised remain far lower, at 5.1%.

The study concluded that direct to consumer advertising has a substantial impact on doctors' prescribing decisions. According to the lead investigator on the study, "A patient request for a specific medication dramatically increases the rate at which physicians prescribe that medication, "These results highlight potential negative impacts of DTC advertising."

One study, from the Journal of General Internal Medicine, found that 57 percent of claims in drug ads were potentially misleading and another 10 percent were just plain lies.

Drug companies are relying more and more heavily on their marketing to American consumers. Last year, the pharmaceutical industry spent $5.2 billion on ads promoting specific drugs—an increase of 16 percent over the previous year.

The American Medical Association has become so concerned about the direct to consumer advertising by pharmaceutical companies that last November is called for an outright ban on such advertising. The money drug companies spend on marketing is far more than the money spent on research. The American Medical Association believes this direct to consumer advertising is fueling the escalating drug prices.

Not only does this marketing raise the cost of our entire healthcare, but it also acts as a form of hidden diagnosis.

Direct to consumer advertising creates in the consumer a fear of an unknown or misunderstood, dangerous enemy, and offers a false solution.

Chapter 35
Time and Money as Barriers to Informed Consent

Being a physician has always been a busy and hectic job. Doctors don't have unlimited time to spend with patients and insurance companies have definite schedules of payment for doctor's visits. According to various studies, doctors spend an average of 15 minutes with each patient. Some physician's who work at hospitals say they've been asked to see patients every 11 minutes.

This time pressure doesn't give a lot of room for physician and patient communication and the adherence to all the steps of Informed Consent required by law.

Rushed doctors listen less -

> *"In the sick room, ten cents' worth of human understanding equals ten dollars' worth of medical science."*
> *- Martin H. Fischer*
> *Physician and Teacher*

A study conducted in 1999 of family physicians found that doctors let patients speak for only 23 seconds before redirecting them.

The same study showed that only one in four patients got to finish their statement.

In 2001 this time was shortened to 12 seconds before the patient was interrupted by the doctor, a beeper, or a knock on the door.

Yet making the patient feel like they have been listened to and understood may be one of the most important parts of doctoring.

Shorter visits place a good deal of strain on the doctor-patient relationship, which is considered a vital ingredient to good medical care. This lack of time, naturally results in less communication and is likely to increase patient frustration. Shorter visits have also been shown to increase the likelihood that the patient will leave with a prescription for medication, rather than a recommendation for a lifestyle change, such as losing weight or beginning an exercise program.

Surveys show doctors are no more happy with this lack of time than are their patients. However, for primary care doctors, time is very literally money. Without the expensive procedures specialists get paid well for performing, and with the limits set by insurance providers, doctors frequently face financial pressures in their practice. This is not to say most family doctors are poor, but they have trained long and hard to be able to provide this vital service to their patients and deserve to be paid well.

But, this need to make a good living should never get in the way of the best practices of medicine.

It's incumbent upon both doctors and their patients to do what they can to stop this slide into shorter and shorter appointments. We must change this system to protect patients and the integrity of the medical field.

According to an article by Jenny Hope for London's Daily Mail, family doctors in Great Britain are demanding an increase in consultation times, claiming currently allowable appointment times are unsafe, putting patients at risk of misdiagnosis or mistakes with their medication.

Until the healthcare system is corrected and doctors schedule more time with each patient, you, as the patient must insist on the right to spend time with your doctor and have the full communication that is your legal right to Informed Consent.

Chapter 36
Physician Concern About Giving Too Much Information

Sometimes doctors worry about giving the patient too much information, especially about dangers and drug side effects. They fear extended explanations may lead to patient refusal to agree to a potentially life-saving treatment.

However, the laws of Informed Consent decrees that patients do have a right to be informed. It should be one of the skills of any doctor to be able to relate information accurately, without frightening the patient.

In some situations, maybe the benefits of a certain treatment don't really outweigh the risks. Doctors must be honest with themselves about this.

Chapter 37
Patients Failing to Know Their Rights

The first thing patients must understand is that Informed Consent is not just a legal or administrative formality. It is an important right that has been unknown by patients and frequently neglected by doctors.

If you didn't before you read this book, you now know that you have a right to be informed and to participate in all decisions regarding your medical care. As much as you demand this right in each medical appointment and with every doctor you see, you'll find improvement in the medical care you receive and in your ability to participate in that care.

"Unless we put medical freedom into the Constitution, the time will come when medicine will organize itself into an undercover dictatorship.

To restrict the art of healing to doctors and deny equal privileges to others will constitute the Bastille of medical science.

All such laws are un-American and despotic."

Benjamin Rush
Physician and Member of the Continental Congress and Signer of the Declaration of Independence

Chapter 38
Patient's Inability to Understand

Patients need to let their doctor know if there is anything about their diagnosis or proposed treatment they don't understand. Physicians try to make themselves understood, but there is no way of them being sure they've done so, without the patient letting them know.

A patient may ask all the questions he or she needs to in order to obtain sufficient understanding to give Informed Consent or informed refusal for any treatment.

Language and cultural barriers can play their part, and sometimes it's best for the practitioner to enlist the aid of a family member or friend of the patient to help them communicate.

Doctors must be honest, perceptive and able communicators. Lack of the exchange of sufficient, comprehensible information recoils badly on both patient and physician.

> **"If you can't explain it simply, you
> don't understand it well enough."
> - Albert Einstein**

Chapter 39
Lack of Patient Participation

Frightened, nervous, or anxious patients may not want to insist on obtaining more information from a doctor on whom they feel their health depends and whom they frequently don't understand. The fact that patients may say they want the doctor to make the decision does not mean they don't want more information; they are just stating the obvious fact that once their consent has been given, the doctor will make the final decision. And doctors need to be aware that patients may feel intimidated or scared and so be less than honest about their real feelings.

Patients are always under an unusual amount of stress during an illness and can experience a wide variety of uncomfortable emotions - anxiety, fear, depression, even anger and exasperation. This stress should never preclude the patient from participating in their own care and receiving the full breakdown of advice in order to give their Informed Consent to any treatment.

Many illnesses, diseases, and emotional and behavioral challenges can be controlled, prevented and overcome by changes in lifestyle. Doctors wise enough to look to these changes as the first recourse for their patients, sometimes face the biggest barrier of all - lack of patient interest and cooperation. Some people would rather take a pill than exercise or control their diet. A physician has a responsibility to patiently explain the benefits of working together to make lifestyle changes and avoid, if possible, more dangerous interventions.

Chapter 40
Is the Doctor Unaware of Alternatives?

Most doctors in general practice and working in hospitals received the bulk of their education years before your current visit. Since that time, much of what they've learned has come from articles (frequently slanted) in their medical journals, continuing education course (often sponsored by medical device and pharmaceutical companies), advertisements, and the visits and lunches offered by drug company representatives. This leads to limited treatment options which itself leads to a gross downplaying of warnings and side effects.

Doctors are not required to take classes in alternative or complementary medical approaches as part of their continuing education. If they were, perhaps physicians would feel more comfortable branching out from treatments that may not be the safest or the most effective for their patients.

An extremely small number of doctors receive continuing education that covers alternative and complementary treatments, even those proven effective against the very problems the doctor runs across daily in practice.

If the only treatment the doctor knows to recommend is not always effective and comes with serious risks, you can see how he or she may not want to explain all the dangers. If the patient then says, "I don't want to take something this risky. What else have you got?" The doctor has nowhere else to go.

Once again, sometimes the best treatment is the current medical approach, but all too often it would be better to search out alternative or complementary treatments instead. If you're bleeding, acupuncture, supplements or physical therapy are unlikely to help. If you have a fever, it's imperative to find the source and prescribe proper medication to bring it down. If the patient has a broken bone, it needs to be set.

However, there are many, many circumstances where the cure is risky and the treatment can recoil badly on the patient.

Anxiety and depression are two frequent complaints for which patients see their general practitioner. The usual treatment for these is one or more drugs, a solution which has proven to be both potentially dangerous and, in many cases, ineffective.

If your doctor is not aware of any alternatives to treat your condition, then it's up to you to judge whether you need to find a doctor better educated in accepted complementary and alternative practices.

Chapter 41
Becoming an Empowered Patient

"The key to patient empowerment is education."
- Carolyn McClanahan, Becoming an Empowered Patient

These few rules will help you get the most out of your doctor's visit and get the proper medical care you need.

Never forget; you deserve and have a legal right to understand all you can about your health and medical choices.

Be prepared for your appointment

Write down how you are doing, the purpose of your appointment, and your current symptoms.

Make a list of anything that is worrying you, and questions you want answered.

Make a list of any medications you're currently taking.

Bring a list of any vitamins, herbs, or other supplements you take.

Bring notes on your current diet (if it seems this may apply)

Bring backup

If your visit is more than just a check-up, bring someone along to help you understand and think with the information you'll be given. If you feel too ill to make your own decisions, bring a family member you trust to help you.

Don't rush

If you know in advance that you have a complicated situation or lots of questions, ask for a longer appointment in advance.

Once there, warn your doctor that you have questions and take your time.

If your doctor begins inching toward the door, ignore it or ask if he or she is in a hurry. Don't be put off. Informed Consent is an ethical part of medical practice and a law.

Keep in mind that you don't have to make a decision right then about any tests or treatment. You can go home and think about it, or get another opinion.

Ask Questions and get comprehensible answers

Ask all the questions you need in order to understand all that's going on. Get the doctor to answer in layperson's terms. And never let yourself feel too embarrassed, shy, or awkward to insist on full understanding.

If the doctor orders testing, ask why

Not all tests are necessary and all medical testing is expensive. If tests are ordered, as the doctor what he or she hopes to discover, and how that will change your treatment plan. (In some cases this is obvious, such as an x-ray to see if you have a broken bone.)

Be wary of medication

If your doctor has prescribed medication, make sure you are told the risks as well as the benefits. How long has it been on the market? Does the doctor have any relationship with the company (lunches, travel, continuing education, speaking or consultant fees)? What are the risks? How long will you need to take it? Is it habit forming or addictive? Are there alternatives?

Ask for alternatives

Complete Informed Consent includes learning about alternatives to any treatment recommendation. Insist on learning about these alternatives. If the doctor doesn't know, then he or she should refer you to someone who does.

What if you do nothing?

Studies have shown, we are a pretty medicalized society. Not all conditions need to be treated immediately. Some go away on their own. Ask your doctor what is likely to happen if you postpone medical intervention and either don't treat the problem at all, or opt for gentler, alternative approaches.

Don't take orders. Insist on participating in your own health care

Ask what you can do; what lifestyle changes you can make that will help. Many diseases are diet and exercise related. If the doctor is not able to furnish you with the education you need in this area, get a referral to a nutritionist, physical therapist, or other specialist who can.

Take notes

You, a friend, or advocate should take notes during your appointment. In some cases, you might ask if the doctor minds your making a recording on your phone. (It's too easy to forget what's been said under the stress of a medical exam and discussion (especially if you're sitting there in that butt-length, silly paper gown.) You can also ask the doctor to give you notes on what was said and any treatment recommendations.

Getting your medical records

You have a legal right to obtain and, if necessary, correct copies of your medical records. Having copies of your medical records can help you understand and manage your health in the way you see fit and to do so according to your own time frame, comfort level and health goals. You can use the information in your records to do your own research and to get second or third opinions from health care professionals you trust.

You can also use the information to track your own vital signs, such as blood pressure and cholesterol. These medical records can also serve to remind you when you're due for your next preventive care checkup.

You should be able to get records pertaining to your physical and your mental health. The exception to this is psychotherapy notes taken by a mental health professional during a conversation. This exception could act as an odd and unknown influence on the way your are treated by medical professionals.

A neighbor of mine, David, who was being treated for advanced skin cancer, told me a story of how his complaints of pain and worry had been for months ignored by various doctors and nurses at different hospitals he went to for diagnosis and treatment. The poor man couldn't understand why his complaints were going unheeded.

Eventually David got hold of *all* his medical records and discovered a notation saying he was "depressed", "bipolar" and "delusional". Apparently during one of his many doctors' visits this diagnosis was placed in his file. With that one notation, all his credibility disappeared. The tone was set before the doctor even entered the examining room. And my neighbor had no idea. It took time and effort, but once he got those records corrected, health practitioners became far more responsive to what he had to say.

If you get your medical record each time you visit a doctor, errors or misunderstandings can be corrected right away and mysteries can be avoided.

By reviewing copies of your records, you can check for errors or omissions and put in corrections where needed. In some situations, this can make a huge difference in obtaining correct and error-free health care.

You don't have to give a reason for wanting your records, but you may have to make your request in writing and pay a minimal copy charge.

Remember, you can get a second opinion

If you find that you and your doctor are just not on the same page, or you have any doubts about your care, get a second opinion.

If your health care provider seems annoyed or is hurried, get another doctor.

If surgery is being recommended

Ask all the questions you can think of. When it comes to informed consent, there is no such thing as a stupid question, or too many questions. You want to get enough information to understand what will happen during the surgery, what recovery will be like and how it will affect your future. You want to feel as certain as possible of your decision to agree to the procedure (or not).

Learn all you can about your surgeon. Ask your primary care doctor, insurance company, and local medical society. Research online. You want your surgeon to be experienced, well respected, and board certified in performing surgery on your specific problem.

Unnecessary medical testing, surgeries and prescribing are far too prevalent in our system of health care, creating soaring costs, increased risks from side effects, medical errors, and other dangers related to over-treating. By being an educated and empowered patient you can reduce these costs and these risks and get the best care possible.

Final Chapter
If Only I'd Asked (The Role and Responsibilities of the Patient)

Do we continue to do what the government, the drug companies, and many doctors are doing and ignore these rights and freedoms? Or do we insist upon our right to act as a respected and informed participant in our medical care?

Having blind faith in our doctors is not fair to the doctor or to ourselves and it certainly has not helped our health care system.

Although a physician is required by law to inform a patient about benefits, risks, and alternative treatments, the patient must also play an active part in the Informed Consent process. Patients must listen to their doctor and ask questions until they feel fully informed and not stop until they do. By asking questions, you may even give your doctor another opportunity to think through your treatment and possibly come up with another solution, if needed.

It takes courage to ask your doctor to fulfill his or her responsibility to fully inform you about any test, diagnosis, prescription or procedure you are being instructed to take. But, when it comes down to it, it's your body, your health, and your future. And if you get too much of a negative reaction, you probably need to get a second opinion.

Ask for a copy of any clinical notes or observations taken by your physician after your visit.

You must play an active role in order to receive high quality health care. It cannot happen without you. The decision to accept (consent to) or refuse to consent to a type of treatment, therapy, or medication is ultimately yours to make.

As part of this process, you need to provide pertinent information to your doctor, including how much you exercise, what kind of food you eat, beverages you drink, the vitamins or other supplements you take.

As a patient, you must listen closely to what your doctor has to say. If you don't understand something, say so. If you need more of an explanation, ask. Make sure your doctor tells you all about the risks associated with the recommended treatment. Know that these risks are real and wouldn't be part of the documentation if they hadn't happened to patients before you.

The better informed you are, the better decisions you'll be able to make about your health. Also, improved communication gets you involved in your own preventive health care.

The practice of medicine has always worked best as a team effort. You and your doctor together are charged with the responsibility of keeping you well.

You may need to educate your doctor in alternatives, you may even need to ask him or her specifically about any side effects of medications or about whether the benefits of a surgical procedure really do outweigh the risks over the long term.

I can't stress enough how important it is to overcome any reluctance or shyness in insisting on full and open communication with your doctor. What you do can have a huge effect on your personal health, your doctor's success rate, and our over-worked and over-burdened health care system.

Informed Consent is the single most powerful tool we have to improve our healthcare system and get the best medical treatment available.

One by one we can make the change we need in our healthcare to the benefit of both ourselves and our doctors.

I'd like to see medical care where physician, patient, and any needed alternative and complementary practitioners worked together for the good of the patient. Where the gap between conventional medicine and other healing arts was not a chasm, but a smooth and well-worn bridge.

In an ideal world you wouldn't have to insist on your right to be fully informed before giving consent, you wouldn't have to worry about whether your doctor has just had lunch with a representative of the company that makes the expensive new pill you have just been prescribed, you wouldn't have to worry about whether your physician is receiving gifts or speaking fees from a company that makes a product he now recommends, you wouldn't have to wonder whether your surgeon is an investor in the company that makes the new knee she's going to be putting in your body.

In this ideal world you would know that every doctor was up on alternatives to help cure or prevent the onset of a condition and who had the versatility and education to help you understand all your options.

It cannot be denied that the American health care system is a business and as such values treatment over prevention, drugs over lifestyle changes, and surgical procedures over alternative forms of care. The end result of this is frequently far from ideal. The patient ends up taking more and more drugs to treat an illness, without ever addressing the root cause.

For example, cardiologists offer guidelines for exercise and diet to address or prevent cardiovascular disease. Diabetes is known to often have its root in poor diet.

Too many doctors reach immediately for the prescription pad rather than taking the time to enlighten their patients on the benefits of lifestyle changes.

We must remain alert and insist on our right to Informed Consent and do our own homework as needed.

My hope is that this book will help us change the old "doctor knows best' view of medical care to an open dialogue approach between patients and their doctors; that it will help ensure each of us, working in partnership with our physicians and other health practitioners, will get the best possible medical care.

Appendix

Ethical Codes and Oaths for the Medical Profession

Ethical codes stressing the importance of a partnership between doctor and patient and a respect for the patient's rights have been in place since the time of Hippocrates.

The Hippocratic Oath - Ancient and Modern

Generally acknowledged as the first set of rules pertaining to Western medicine, this guide to conduct in the medical profession, first written down over 2500 years ago, is credited to Hippocrates, the "Father of Western Medicine". It's one of the oldest binding documents in recorded history.

The oath has been rewritten many times over the years to keep pace with changes in societal views. For instance, the original Hippocratic oath prohibits physician assisted suicide or abortion. The current version does not contain these restrictions.

Although it's unfortunately no longer considered binding, a pledge to the traditional version or, more frequently a modern rewrite, is part of the graduation ceremonies of many medical schools. Other schools will have students swear to uphold the Declaration of Geneva or the International Code of Medical Ethics.

Here's a translation of the original Hippocratic oath and below it, one of the accepted modern versions.

Although this code is not legally binding, most physicians have sworn to uphold these principles or similar ones as stated in other oaths, as part of their medical school graduation. Understanding these concepts offers an idea of the mindset that physicians are expected to hold.

(If you find words in this document that you don't understand, please take a look at the glossary.)

Classic Version of the Hippocratic Oath Translated From the Greek

I swear by Apollo Physician and Asclepius and Hygieia and Panaceia and all the gods and goddesses, making them my witnesses, that I will fulfill according to my ability and judgment this oath and this covenant:

To hold him who has taught me this art as equal to my parents and to live my life in partnership with him, and if he is in need of money to give him a share of mine, and to regard his offspring as equal to my brothers in male lineage and to teach them this art - if they desire to learn it - without fee and covenant; to give a share of precepts and oral instruction and all the other learning to my sons and to the sons of him who has instructed me and to pupils who have signed the covenant and have taken an oath according to the medical law, but no one else.

I will apply dietetic measures for the benefit of the sick according to my ability and judgment; I will keep them from harm and injustice.

I will neither give a deadly drug to anybody who asked for it, nor will I make a suggestion to this effect. Similarly I will not give to a woman an abortive remedy. In purity and holiness I will guard my life and my art.

I will not use the knife, not even on sufferers from stone, but will withdraw in favor of such men as are engaged in this work.

Whatever houses I may visit, I will come for the benefit of the sick, remaining free of all intentional injustice, of all mischief and in particular of sexual relations with both female and male persons, be they free or slaves.

What I may see or hear in the course of the treatment or even outside of the treatment in regard to the life of men, which on no account one must spread abroad, I will keep to myself, holding such things shameful to be spoken about.

If I fulfill this oath and do not violate it, may it be granted to me to enjoy life and art, being honored with fame among all men for all time to come; if I transgress it and swear falsely, may the opposite of all this be my lot.

From The Hippocratic Oath: Text, Translation, and Interpretation, by Ludwig Edelstein. Baltimore: The Johns Hopkins Press, 1943.

> ***"I will not be ashamed to say, 'I know not' nor will I fail to call in my colleagues when the skills of another are needed for a patient's recovery."***
> ***- Hippocrates***

Modern Version of the Hippocratic Oath

I swear to fulfill, to the best of my ability and judgment, this covenant:

I will respect the hard-won scientific gains of those physicians in whose steps I walk, and gladly share such knowledge as is mine with those who are to follow.

I will apply, for the benefit of the sick, all measures which are required, avoiding those twin traps of overtreatment and therapeutic nihilism.

I will remember that there is art to medicine as well as science, and that warmth, sympathy, and understanding may outweigh the surgeon's knife or the chemist's drug.

I will not be ashamed to say "I know not," nor will I fail to call in my colleagues when the skills of another are needed for a patient's recovery.

I will respect the privacy of my patients, for their problems are not disclosed to me that the world may know. Most especially must I tread with care in matters of life and death. If it is given me to save a life, all thanks. But it may also be within my power to take a life; this awesome responsibility must be faced with great humbleness and awareness of my own frailty. Above all, I must not play at God.

I will remember that I do not treat a fever chart, a cancerous growth, but a sick human being, whose illness may affect the person's family and economic stability. My responsibility includes these related problems, if I am to care adequately for the sick.

I will prevent disease whenever I can, for prevention is preferable to cure.

I will remember that I remain a member of society, with special obligations to all my fellow human beings, those sound of mind and body as well as the infirm.

If I do not violate this oath, may I enjoy life and art, respected while I live and remembered with affection thereafter. May I always act so as to preserve the finest traditions of my calling and may I long experience the joy of healing those who seek my help.

Written in 1964 by Louis Lasagna, Academic Dean of the School of Medicine at Tufts University, and used in many medical schools today.

World Medical Association, Declaration of Geneva

Likely in response to the atrocities committed by doctors in Nazi concentration camps, in 1948, the 2nd General Assembly of the World Medical Association adopted the Declaration of Geneva. This declaration was amended in 1968 and again in 1983, 1994, 2005, 2006.

Administered at the time of being admitted as a member of the medical profession. (Currently used by many schools in Europe and the United States)

I solemnly pledge to consecrate my life to the service of humanity;

I will give to my teachers the respect and gratitude which is their due;

I will practice my profession with conscience and dignity;

The health of my patient will be my first consideration;

I will respect the secrets which are confided in me, even after the patient has died;

I will maintain by all means in my power, the honor and the noble traditions of the medical profession;

My colleagues will be my brothers;

I will not permit considerations of religion, nationality, race, party politics, or social standing to intervene between my duty and my patient;
I will maintain the utmost respect for human life from its beginning even under threat and I will not use my medical knowledge contrary to the laws of humanity;

I make these promises solemnly, freely, and upon my honor.

World Medical Association International Code of Medical Ethics

Adopted by the 3rd General Assembly of the World Medical Association, London, England, October 1949 and amended by the 22nd World Medical Assembly Sydney, Australia, August 1968 and the 35th World Medical Assembly Venice, Italy, October 1983 and the 57th WMA General Assembly, Pilanesberg, South Africa, October 2006

This is the latest version, taken from the WMA Website.

Duties of Physicians in General

A physician shall always exercise his/her independent professional judgment and maintain the highest standards of professional conduct.

A physician shall respect a competent patient's right to accept or refuse treatment.

A physician shall not allow his/her judgment to be influenced by personal profit or unfair discrimination.

A physician shall be dedicated to providing competent medical service in full professional and moral independence, with compassion and respect for human dignity.

A physician shall deal honestly with patients and colleagues, and report to the appropriate authorities those physicians who practice unethically or incompetently or who engage in fraud or deception.

A physician shall not receive any financial benefits or other incentives solely for referring patients or prescribing specific products.

A physician shall respect the rights and preferences of patients, colleagues, and other health professionals.

A physician shall recognize his/her important role in educating the public but should use due caution in divulging discoveries or new techniques or treatment through non-professional channels.

A physician shall certify only that which he/she has personally verified.

A physician shall strive to use health care resources in the best way to benefit patients and their community.

A physician shall seek appropriate care and attention if he/she suffers from mental or physical illness.

A physician shall respect the local and national codes of ethics.

Duties of Physicians to Patients

A physician shall always bear in mind the obligation to respect human life.

A physician shall act in the patient's best interest when providing medical care.

A physician shall owe his/her patients complete loyalty and all the scientific resources available to him/her. Whenever an examination or treatment is beyond the physician's capacity, he/she should consult with or refer to another physician who has the necessary ability.

A physician shall respect a patient's right to confidentiality. It is ethical to disclose confidential information when the patient consents to it or when there is a real and imminent threat of harm to the patient or to others and this threat can be only removed by a breach of confidentiality.

A physician shall give emergency care as a humanitarian duty unless he/she is assured that others are willing and able to give such care.

A physician shall in situations when he/she is acting for a third party, ensure that the patient has full knowledge of that situation.

A physician shall not enter into a sexual relationship with his/her current patient or into any other abusive or exploitative relationship.

Duties of Physicians to Colleagues

A physician shall behave towards colleagues as he/she would have them behave towards him/her.

A physician shall not undermine the patient-physician relationship of colleagues in order to attract patients.

A physician shall when medically necessary, communicate with colleagues who are involved in the care of the same patient. This communication should respect patient confidentiality and be confined to necessary information.

> *"A physician shall respect the rights and preferences of patients, colleagues, and other health professionals."*
> *- World Medical Association*
> *International Code of Medical Ethics*

Patient's Bill of Rights (American Hospital Association)

Here you will find a summary of the Consumer Bill of Rights and Responsibilities that was adopted by the US Advisory Commission on Consumer Protection and Quality in the Health Care Industry in 1998. It is also known as the Patient's Bill of Rights.

The initial Patient's Bill of Rights was established in 1973 by the American Hospital Association, AHA. It was then revised by the AHA in 1992 to include additional rights and better define the details of all patients' rights.

The Patient's Bill of Rights was created to try to reach 3 major goals:

1. To help patients feel more confident in the US health care system; the Bill of Rights:

• Assures that the health care system is fair and it works to meet patients' needs

• Gives patients a way to address any problems they may have

• Encourages patients to take an active role in staying or getting healthy

2. To stress the importance of a strong relationship between patients and their   health care providers

3. To stress the key role patients play in staying healthy by laying out rights and responsibilities for all patients and health care providers

This Bill of Rights also applies to the insurance plans offered to federal employees. Many other health insurance plans and facilities have also adopted these values. Even Medicare and Medicaid stand by many of them.

The 8 key areas of the Patient's Bill of Rights

<u>Information for patients</u>

You have the right to accurate and easily understood information about your health plan, health care professionals, and health care facilities. If you speak another language, have a physical or mental disability, or just don't understand something, help should be given so you can make informed health care decisions.

<u>Choice of providers and plans</u>

You have the right to choose health care providers who can give you high-quality health care when you need it.

<u>Access to emergency services</u>
If you have severe pain, an injury, or sudden illness that makes you believe that your health is in danger, you have the right to be screened and stabilized using emergency services.

You should be able to use these services whenever and wherever you need them, without needing to wait for authorization and without any financial penalty.

<u>Taking part in treatment decisions</u>

You have the right to know your treatment options and take part in decisions about your care.

Parents, guardians, family members, or others that you choose can speak for you if you cannot make your own decisions.

Respect and non-discrimination

You have a right to considerate, respectful care from your doctors, health plan representatives, and other health care providers that does not discriminate against you.

Confidentiality (privacy) of health information

You have the right to talk privately with health care providers and to have your health care information protected. You also have the right to read and copy your own medical record. You have the right to ask that your doctor change your record if it is not correct, relevant, or complete.

Complaints and appeals

You have the right to a fair, fast, and objective review of any complaint you have against your health plan, doctors, hospitals or other health care personnel. This includes complaints about waiting times, operating hours, the actions of health care personnel, and the adequacy of health care facilities.

Consumer responsibilities

In a health care system that protects consumer or patients' rights, patients should expect to take on some responsibilities to get well and/or stay well (for instance, exercising and not using tobacco). Patients are expected to do things like treat health care workers and other patients with respect, try to pay their medical bills, and follow the rules and benefits of their health plan coverage. Having patients involved in their care increases the chance of the best possible outcomes and helps support a high quality, cost-conscious health care system.

Health insurance problems

If you have concerns about your insurance, it is sometimes helpful to start with customer service or a case manager at your health insurance company.

Patients' Bill of Rights (Association of American Physicians and Surgeons)

In 1995 the Association of American Physicians and Surgeons, AAPS, adopted its own **Patient Bill of Rights**, termed "freedoms" that state the groups' stand on protocols between physicians and patients and also between physicians, patients and health insurance plans.

All patients should be guaranteed the following freedoms:

To seek consultation with the physician(s) of their choice;

To contract with their physician(s) on mutually agreeable terms;

To be treated confidentially, with access to their records limited to those involved in their care or designated by the patient;

To use their own resources to purchase the care of their choice;

To refuse medical treatment even if it is recommended by their physician(s);

To be informed about their medical condition, the risks and benefits of treatment and appropriate alternatives;

To refuse third-party interference in their medical care, and to be confident that their actions in seeking or declining medical care will not result in third-party-imposed penalties for patients or physicians;

To receive full disclosure of their insurance plan in plain language, including:

Contracts: A copy of the contract between the physician and health care plan, and between the patient or employer and the plan;

Incentives: Whether participating physicians are offered financial incentives to reduce treatment or ration care;

Cost: The full cost of the plan, including copayments, coinsurance, and deductibles;

Coverage: Benefits covered and excluded, including availability and location of 24-hour emergency care;

Qualifications: A roster and qualifications of participating physicians;

Approval Procedures: Authorization procedures for services, whether doctors need approval of a committee or any other individual, and who decides what is medically necessary;

Referrals: Procedures for consulting a specialist, and who must authorize the referral;

Appeals: Grievance procedures for claim or treatment denials;

Gag Rule: Whether physicians are subject to a gag rule, preventing criticism of the plan.

Principles of Medical Ethics
American Medical Association

Preamble

The medical profession has long subscribed to a body of ethical statements developed primarily for the benefit of the patient. As a member of this profession, a physician must recognize responsibility to patients first and foremost, as well as to society, to other health professionals, and to self. The following Principles adopted by the American Medical Association are not laws, but standards of conduct which define the essentials of honorable behavior for the physician.

Principles of medical ethics

I. A physician shall be dedicated to providing competent medical care, with compassion and respect for human dignity and rights.

II. A physician shall uphold the standards of professionalism, be honest in all professional interactions, and strive to report physicians deficient in character or competence, or engaging in fraud or deception, to appropriate entities.

III. A physician shall respect the law and also recognize a responsibility to seek changes in those requirements which are contrary to the best interests of the patient.

IV. A physician shall respect the rights of patients, colleagues, and other health professionals, and shall safeguard patient confidences and privacy within the constraints of the law.

V. A physician shall continue to study, apply, and advance scientific knowledge, maintain a commitment to medical education, make relevant information available to patients, colleagues, and the public, obtain consultation, and use the talents of other health professionals when indicated.

VI. A physician shall, in the provision of appropriate patient care, except in emergencies, be free to choose whom to serve, with whom to associate, and the environment in which to provide medical care.

VII. A physician shall recognize a responsibility to participate in activities contributing to the improvement of the community and the betterment of public health.

VIII. A physician shall, while caring for a patient, regard responsibility to the patient as paramount.

IX. A physician shall support access to medical care for all people.

Adopted June 1957; revised June 1980; revised June 2001.

"A physician shall continue to study, apply and advance scientific knowledge, maintain a commitment to medical education, make relevant information available to patients, colleagues, and the public, obtain consultation, and use the talents of other health professionals when indicated."
- Principles of Medical Ethics
American Medical Association

Basic Steps of Informed Consent (AMA)

The Law Regarding Informed Consent Requires the Physician (not a Delegated Representative) Disclose and Discuss With the Patient the Following:

The diagnosis, if known

The nature and purpose of a proposed treatment or procedure

The risks and benefits of proposed treatment or procedures

Alternatives (regardless of costs or extent covered by insurance)

The risks and benefits of alternatives

The risks and benefits of not receiving treatments or undergoing procedures

Source: American Medical Association

Graphs and Charts

Countries in Order of Longest Life Span

Rank	Country	Yrs	Rank	Country	Yrs
1	Monaco	89.52	26	Cayman Isle	81.13
2	Japan	84.74	27	Isle of Man	81.09
3	Singapore	84.68	28	New Zealand	81.05
4	Macau	84.51	29	Belgium	80.88
5	San Marino	83.24	30	Finland	80.77
6	Iceland	82.97	31	Ireland	80.68
7	Hong Kong	82.86	32	Germany	80.57
8	Andorra	82.72	33	United Kingdom	80.54
9	Switzerland	82.50	34	Greece	80.43
10	Guernsey	82.47	35	Saint Pierre	80.39
11	Israel	82.27	36	Malta	80.25
12	Luxembourg	82.17	37	Faroe Islands	80.24
13	Australia	82.15	38	E.U.	80.20
14	Italy	82.12	39	Korea, South	80.04
15	Sweden	81.98	40	Taiwan	79.98
16	Liechtenstein	81.77	41	Virgin Islands	79.89
17	Jersey	81.76	42	Turks	79.69
18	Canada	81.76	43	United States	79.68
19	France	81.75	44	Wallis & Futuna	79.57
20	Norway	81.70	45	Saint Helena	79.36
21	Spain	81.57	46	Gibraltar	79.28
22	Austria	81.39	47	Denmark	79.25
23	Anguilla	81.31	48	Puerto Rico	79.25

24	Netherlands	81.23		49	Portugal	79.16
25	Bermuda	81.15		50	Guam	78.98

Countries Spending the Most on Healthcare
Per Capita Health Care Costs

#1	United States	$8,713
#2	Switzerland	$6,325
#3	Sweden	$4,904
#4	Germany	$4,819
#5	Canada	$4,351
#6	France	$4,124
#7	Australia	$3,866
#8	Japan	$3,713
#9	United Kingdom	$3,235
#10	Italy	$3,077

**Pharmaceutical Company Spending
R & D Versus Advertising
(2013)**

**Advertising
$98.3 Billion**

**R & D
$65.8 Billion**

Sometime pharmaceutical companies argue they need to charge such high prices for drugs in order to finance Research and Discovery (R & D) for new drugs. However, here we see how much pharmaceutical manufacturers spend on marketing vs. advertising.

Most of this marketing money is directed at the physicians who do the prescribing.

In 2012 drug companies spend $2 Billion marketing to consumers in the U.S. and an estimated $24 billion marketing directly to health care professionals.

Death by Medical Error

Death in the United States

Johns Hopkins University researchers estimate that medical error is now the third leading cause of death. Here's a ranking by yearly deaths.

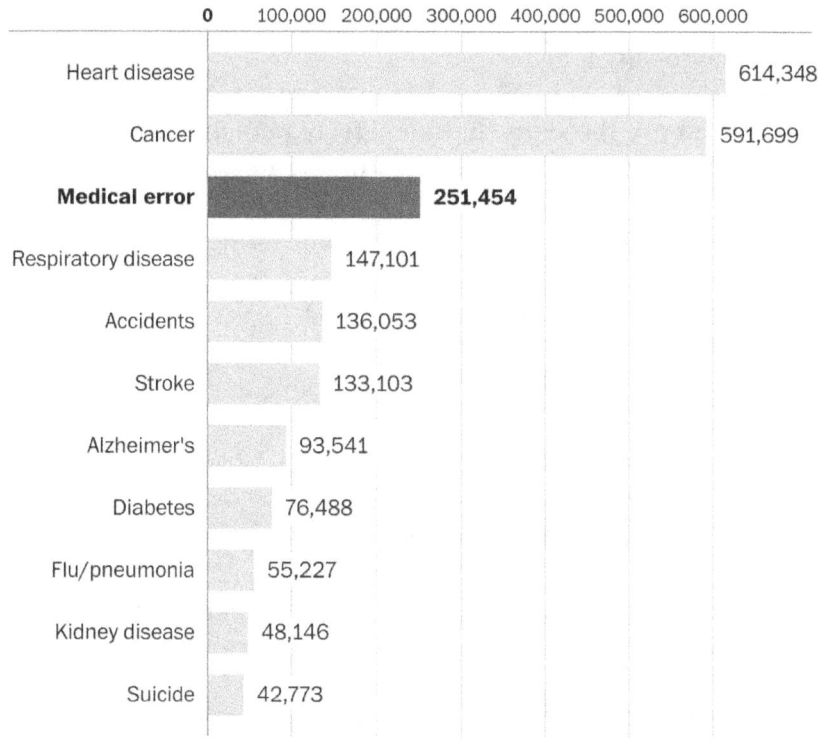

Heart disease	614,348
Cancer	591,699
Medical error	**251,454**
Respiratory disease	147,101
Accidents	136,053
Stroke	133,103
Alzheimer's	93,541
Diabetes	76,488
Flu/pneumonia	55,227
Kidney disease	48,146
Suicide	42,773

Source: National Center for Health Statistics, BMJ

THE WASHINGTON POST

Interview with Donna Rybacki
Senior Care Specialist and Advocate for Senior Rights

How did you decide to become involved in helping seniors?

I was a school teacher for 22 years while raising a family of 6. I gained a lot of experience dealing with families and their interactions. I like to help, guide and mentor. I have been successful in helping families work together in tough times and become problem solvers together. This profession seemed to be an excellent place for me to utilize all of my skills and knowledge to help families move through a transition that can be very emotionally tough.

What are the signs that an elderly person may need assistance and guidance in making healthcare decisions?

When there are noticeable signs such as these:

Is their personal hygiene declining?

Does it seem as if they may not be able to care for those needs?

Is he or she not eating properly?

Do they seem undernourished?

Are they declining family get-togethers and other social activities they once loved?

Are they not able to properly manage their medications?

Are there signs of memory loss and is it worsening?

Do they seem frail and at risk of falling?

Are they at risk for falling victim to crime?

Usually you will also notice that they are making excuses for the neglect of these usually normal functions.

What should a family member do when they begin to see these signs?

When these signs are present, the first thing the family members should do is to take the time to really observe without getting overtly invasive, which could frighten them or cause them to create a social screen to keep you away, and see if they just need a little more help now.

Next, make that appointment with their primary care physician to see if there are any health changes that need to be addressed.

Set up a plan of action with other family members to "check-in" more to make sure things are going well and if they are declining take the necessary steps to put in a healthy care plan whether at home or if appropriate in an assisted living environment where they have care staff on site for their needs.

What are some of the things an advocate for an elderly relation needs to be aware of when ensuring their relation does not get pushed into treatments that may not be in the patient's best interest?

The first thing is to *BE* AWARE; just because an elderly person is in a hospital or other medical or licensed care facility short term or long term does not mean that the staff at that institution KNOWS the residents/patients' rights.

Stay connected to the situation and ask questions about the proposed treatments, especially if they include drugs or any kind, especially psychoactive drugs. Look these drugs up and see what they are designed for and if it seems like it will help the situation; many times, if it is a psychiatric drug being prescribed for treatment, it is just to temporarily calm a situation and in the long run may be very harmful. Find out exactly what it is and make sure that it is in the best interest of the patient to allow it.

I observe more times than not that neither the resident nor the family members realize their right to informed consent and the right to refuse treatments. Many times where the elderly person is concerned some treatments get done before the family member is even informed of the need for a change of care plan.

How can an advocate or guardian help make sure their loved one is not being unnecessarily drugged?

If your elderly loved one lives alone make sure that at their home there is an advanced care directive that states NO DRUGGING OR TREATMENT WITHOUT CONSENT and that this directive is near the door or a place where an emergency response team or paramedic can easily see it if there is an accident or emergency. Do not leave it in a file or drawer; it may not be found.

Additionally, if they have dementia then add the statement:

NO DRUGGING OR TREATMENT WITHOUT CONSENT OF THE FAMILY MEMBER, OR AGENT PRESENT.

The doctors are obligated to respect that; it doesn't mean that they may not try to ignore it but it is not legal to override that document.

Keep close eye on things so that you can notice any change in behavior or condition. Make sure if your loved one is in a care facility that the people at the facility are aware that they DO NOT have your permission to add any dosage, or any medication to the routine unless you are aware and approve.

Recently a family member called me for help; her mother was in a residential care home where she had been living happily for two years. The daughter was concerned because she said the last time she visited her mom she was very lethargic, could hardly move and looked almost comatose. She could not speak her needs only calling out "help me".

In talking to the care staff she found out that a medication that was PRN (abbreviation meaning "when necessary") only was increased to be given on a regular routine now three times a day. The care staff and the administrator went ahead and asked the doctor who was a house call doctor at the home to increase this and they did without the daughter's consent. It took the daughter three weeks to undo this "order" which was not authorized. Once they reduced the amount, her mom was no longer comatose and was *almost* back to the way she was before the over medicating.

What advice do you have for family members charged with the responsibility of making decisions for elderly relatives who have become unable to make informed health decisions on their own?

Make sure that you get these questions answered by the physician before any treatment is administered.

1. The reason for the particular drug;
2. The medical condition for which the drug is needed;
3. How long and how often the drug will be used;
4. How the resident's medical condition will be affected;
5. The nature, degree, duration and probability of known side effects;
6. The reasonable alternative treatments.

Keep in mind the resident's right to accept or refuse the psychoactive drug and, if he or she consents, they have the right to revoke consent for any reason at any time.

Federal guidelines state that <u>*antipsychotic drugs should not be used*</u> if the only symptoms are:

wandering
unsociability
poor self-care
inattention or indifference to surroundings
restlessness
fidgeting
impaired memory
nervousness
mild anxiety
uncooperativeness
insomnia
behavior that does not represent a danger to others

Many antipsychotic and anti-anxiety drugs used to treat residents with dementia are both not medically indicated and a form of chemical restraint. I believe that it is happening too much in the assisted living arena as well as nursing homes where there are elderly people.

Is there anything else you'd like to mention regarding the law of Informed Consent and its application to seniors and the elderly?

I recommend anyone who has an elderly relative read the following, and other information available on the CANHR website:

This information is provided by CANHR article on *TOXIC MEDICINE http://canhr.org/*

The information part of informed consent requires doctors to explain any proposed treatment to their patients and, if applicable, to their patients' legal representatives.

The consent part of informed consent simply requires that patients or their representatives agree to any form of health care treatment before it is undertaken. Failure to obtain consent before administering treatment is battery against the patient.

The key informed consent regulations are found at sections 72528 and 72527(a)(4) &(5) of Title 22 of the California Code of Regulations.

See the Laws and Regulations section on page 18 for a complete listing of pertinent laws and regulations.

Donna Rybacki
Senior Care Specialist
American Senior Home Finders
AmericanSeniorHomeFinders.com

A Look at Informed Consent
By Tony Chicotel
Attorney / Advocate

Informed consent is both a legal and medical concept, making the patient the ultimate decision-maker regarding all important decisions concerning health. Informed consent has two parts:

1) consent, meaning all decisions regarding a patient's proposed health care treatments require his or her consent and

2) informed, meaning the patient must be told by his or her physician the benefits, risks, and alternatives to all proposed treatments.

A host of state and federal laws defining and protecting patients' rights to give or withhold informed consent ensure that patients control their bodies and their health care treatments.

Physicians provide guidance and recommendations, patients make choices.

The necessity of patient consent was largely borne of American "case law" meaning law developed by judges as they ruled on court cases brought before them. In these first informed consent cases, patients who had treatments or procedures done to them without their knowledge or consent sued the health care provider for subsequent injuries. The court's anchored their decisions in favor of the patients in American notions of autonomy: the right of patients to control what happens to their bodies. As the people who, by far, stand the most to gain or lose regarding health care decisions, patients are best suited to make those decisions.

Once the law had clarified that patient consent is required before a health care provider can initiate treatment, additional cases addressed the physician's duty to inform the patient regarding risks, benefits, and alternatives.

While the patients decide, their physicians are obligated to do their best to ensure those decisions are informed and therefore must explain the important factors to consider. The extent of the information that must be communicated to patients varies from state to state and, sometimes, from procedure to procedure, but generally must include everything that is important, including risks, benefits, and alternatives.

For older adults, informed consent is particularly important.

Older adults, on average, have more health care interventions and thus may have more to consider, especially regarding how different interventions work with one another. Additionally, some older adults may be more deferential to physician recommendations and less willing to control their own health care decisions. Finally, older adults have to be especially careful to make sure their physicians are disclosing all care options. Bias against older adults or even financial pressures to limit health care costs within a managed care system may inhibit physicians from raising expensive or riskier treatment options as they worry about the potential "futility" of expending resources when the expected life span will not be significantly lengthened.

People with cognitive disabilities have special considerations regarding informed consent. If their disabilities preclude them from being able to appreciate risks, benefits, and alternatives, consent must be obtained from a legally authorized surrogate, or substitute, decision-maker.

In some cases, the patient may have a court-appointed guardian or an agent named in a power of attorney or advance health care directive. In other cases, state law or common practice may allow a spouse, partner, family member, or friend to serve as a surrogate.

The key is that physicians or other health care providers are usually excluded from acting as surrogates and not permitted to accept or decline health care interventions on behalf of their patients.

The corollary to the right to informed consent is the right to refuse. Other than patients who have been found to be legally unable to make their own health care decisions, all patients have the right to refuse any treatment regardless of how necessary their physicians believe it to be.

Case Study - psychotropic drugs

Psychotropic drugs are used to alter a patient's thinking, mood, or behavior. Almost by definition, psychotropics are given to patients who are believed to have problems with thinking and therefore, may be potentially unable to make decisions about their health care treatment. Because of the association of psychotropics with impaired thinking, patients are often deprived of their rights regarding informed consent before taking them. Their physicians figure the mental impairment renders informed consent issues moot.

However, as previously mentioned patients always have the right to provide informed consent unless they have delegated it to a surrogate and they always have the right to withhold consent unless a court has determined the patient lacks the capacity to do so.

Psychotropics are associated with a number of risks, particularly for older adults, and in some contexts in which they are frequently prescribed, are often ineffective at improving quality of life. It is important for patients and their representatives to make sure their right informed consent is acknowledged and honored in all health care contexts.

Tony Chicotel
Attorney/Advocate for Residents of Long-term Care Facilities

A Patient's Rights Attorney Discusses Informed Consent

When healthcare is provided, the practitioner is required to obtain the informed consent of the patient, with limited exceptions. The specific definition of informed consent may vary from state to state, yet it basically means that a healthcare provider must tell a patient all of the potential benefits, risks and alternatives involved in any procedure or course of treatment and must obtain the patient's written consent to proceed.

This principle is based upon the patient being in control of his or her own health decisions, no matter how difficult, and that the patient trusts the healthcare provider to tell all.

The point is that while the physician or other healthcare practitioner may have vast knowledge and draw upon a great deal of history about the patient, they cannot usurp the right of the patient to evaluate their own situation and determine the path they want to follow.

If the healthcare provider fails to follow this fundamental rule of practice they may be held responsible by a court of law and by their governing state board or department.

The doctrine of informed consent is a vital central rule of ethics in the healing arts supported by laws developed over the centuries. Applied to medical research due to the Nuremberg investigations about torture, a code was developed making it significantly wrong to experiment on incarcerated humans unless and until their individual rights are respected. This idea was further reinforced by the Declaration of Helsinki.

Yet neither was codified in law, so California passed a series of statutes in the Health and Safety Code at sections 24170 through 24179.5. Yet experimentation continues to this day without respect for these rules of laws and doctrines developed before them.

California has a Code of Regulations in which the requirement to provide informed consent in psychotherapeutic matters is specified at 22 CCR § 72528.

In over thirty years applied to this area of law I have never seen it applied.

The California Hospital Association has a Consent Manual explaining patients' rights.

In California there are claims that can be pursued in civil courts upon a theory that informed consent was not provided. The jury instruction (CACI 532) provides that a medical procedure cannot be performed unless and until the patient has provided an informed consent.

While the jury instruction does not specifically state it, the practitioner is supposed to supply the patient with other options even if not recommended by the advising practitioner. This last point is continuously ignored. The failure to obtain informed consent is alone a basis for a civil remedy.

Consider the application of this vital doctrine to elder care, where quality of life and end of life decisions must be confronted. Skilled care facility nurses and physicians must be specially trained for these events and providing the information to the elderly or their families is vital.

I implore the public to undertake independent research and ask questions.

Gary S. Brown
Patient's Right Attorney
Civil Trial Specialist

Glossary

adverse event, an adverse event is any undesirable experience associated with the use of a medical product in a patient.

advocate, (n) someone who fights for something or someone, especially someone who fights for the rights of others or another. (v) to speak, write or stand up for something or someone.

alternative, an additional choice

alternative medicine, complementary and integrative medicine, also called alternative medicine; includes treatments that are not part of mainstream medicine.

AMA, American Medical Association

American Medical Association, founded in 1847, the American Medical Association is the largest association of physicians; MDs, DOs, and medical students.

anticholineric (side effect), anticholinergic side effects may place patients, particularly older patients, in a position to suffer from serious medical complications

Apollo Physician, one of the gods Hippocrates swears by in his famous oath, Apollo is the ancient Greek and Roman god of light, healing, music, poetry, prophecy, and manly beauty.

arrhythmia, abnormal or irregular heartbeat

Asclepius, this god, mentioned by Hippocrates, is one of the earliest Greek gods to specialize in healing. Healers and those in need of healing invoked Asclepius' name in prayer and healing ceremonies in temples and at home. A healing clan known as the Asclepiads claimed to be the descendants of Asclepius and to have inherited a knowledge and mystical power of healing from him.

battery, if a doctor treats a patient without that patient's Informed Consent this is legally considered battery, no matter how skillfully the treatment was done. This is because a medical treatment involves touching a patient, and *battery* is defined as "unconsented to touching".

Bell's palsy, a condition that causes a temporary weakness or paralysis of the muscles in the face

benefit, anything that promotes well-being, an advantage

Bill of Rights, list of the most important rights given to a particular situation or group

Black Box Warning, this type of warning the may appear on a prescription drug's label and is designed to call attention to serious or life-threatening risks.

CAM, initial used for the umbrella grouping of complementary and alternative medicine

One of the most widely accepted definitions of complementary and alternative medicine comes from David Eisenberg, MD, director of Complementary and Integrative Medical Therapies at Harvard University:

"Complementary and alternative medicine are those practices explicitly used for medical intervention, health promotion, or disease prevention which are not routinely taught at United States medical schools, nor routinely underwritten by third party payers within the existing United States health care system."

The National Center for Complementary and Alternative Medicine (NCCAM) defines complementary and alternative medicine in a similar way, as "a group of diverse medical and health care systems, practices, and products that are not presently considered to be part of conventional medicine."

cardiac neurosis, (a kind of anxiety in which the person experiences quick fatigue, shortness of breath, rapid heart beat, dizziness and other cardiac (heart) symptoms, but not caused by heart disease

complementary medicine, non-conventional medicine, when it is used together with conventional medicine

consent, to permit, approve, or agree; (n) permission, approval, agreement, or compliance

conventional medicine, medicine as usually practiced by holders of M.D. (medical doctor) or D.O. (doctor of osteopathic medicine) degrees and by their allied health professionals such as physical therapists and registered nurses

covenant, an agreement, usually formal, between two or more persons to do or not do something specified.

delirium, a serious disturbance in mental abilities that results in confused thinking and reduced awareness of your environment

diabetic neuropathy, diabetic neuropathy is a type of nerve damage that can occur if you have diabetes.

dietetic, relating to diet or adapted for use in special diets; (n) the science concerned with the nutritional planning and preparation of foods

DO, Doctor of Osteopathy, according to the American Osteopathic Association, Doctors of Osteopathic Medicine, or DOs, are fully licensed physicians who practice in all areas of medicine. Emphasizing a whole-person approach to treatment and care, DOs are trained to listen and partner with their patients to help them get healthy and stay well.

fibromyalgia, a chronic physical condition commonly characterized by widespread muscle pain, fatigue, concentration issues, and sleep problems

freedoms, not having external control, interference, or regulation - the power to determine action without restraint.

gout, a type of painful arthritis

GSK, abbreviation for drug manufacturer GlaxoSmithKline

Hippocratic oath, an oath, or pledge attributed to Hippocrates, but possibly written by a contemporary of his that serves as an ethical guide for the medical profession. The original Hippocratic oath or a modern version is incorporated into the graduation ceremonies of many medical colleges.

holistic, dealing with or treating the whole of something or someone and not just a parts

Hygieia; the goddess of good health, one of the Greek gods and goddesses mentioned in the original version of the Hippocratic Oath. She was the daughter of Asclepius and a companion of Aphrodite. Her sisters included Panacea (cure-all) and Iaso (remedy). She was the goddess of welfare and prevention of disease.

The English word *hygiene,* meaning; clean or healthy practices or the science concerned with the maintenance of health is derived from the name of this goddess.

inform, to give information; supply knowledge or enlightenment

informed, having or prepared with information or knowledge

Informed Consent, by law, your health care providers must explain your health condition and treatment choices to you. This is Informed Consent.

integrative medicine, integrative medicine is the term used for bringing conventional and complementary approaches together in a coordinated way. The use of integrative approaches to health and wellness has grown within care settings across the United States. Researchers are currently exploring the potential benefits of integrative health in a variety of situations, including pain management for military personnel and veterans, relief of symptoms in cancer patients and survivors, and programs to promote healthy behaviors.

internist, a physician specializing in the diagnosis and nonsurgical treatment of diseases, especially of adults.

lymphedema, lymphedema is swelling in the arms and legs that is stemming from the lymphatic system. A trained PT can perform certain types of lymphatic drainage massage or use other techniques to help decrease swelling in a limb.
medical ethics, a set of beliefs about right and wrong in the field of medicine. Medical ethics aren't the same as laws, which are strict rules, enforceable by state or local governments and the Justice system. Informed Consent is enforceable by law, whereas other medical codes, such as the Hippocratic oath are ethical standards. Ethics play a vital part in the practice of medicine.

neurodermatitis, a skin condition that starts with a patch of itchy skin. Scratching makes it even itchier

Panaceia; name of a Greek goddess mentioned in the original Hippocratic Oath. In Greek mythology Panaceia was the goddess of healing and cures. She was the daughter of Asclepius, god of healing and medicine and granddaughter of Apollo, god of healing.

The English word *panacea*, meaning; a cure-all or remedy for all disease or ills comes from the name of this goddess.
peripheral neuropathy, pain, numbness, tingling or burning sensation that occurs in the hands, feet or legs

pathologize, the practice of seeing a symptom as indication of a disease or disorder. In mental health, the term is often used to indicate over-diagnosis or the refusal to accept certain behavior as normal.

polyphenols, a kind of chemical that (at least in theory) may protect against some common health problems and possibly certain effects of aging risk, exposure the chance of injury or loss

sacroiliac joint, the sacroiliac joints are located at the bottom of the back. You have one either side of the spine.)
sciatica, a medical condition of pain going down the leg from the lower back. This pain may go down the back, outside, or front of the leg)

side effects, any effect of a drug, chemical, or other medicine that is additional to its intended effect, especially an effect that is harmful, dangerous, or unpleasant

tardive dyskinesia, involuntary, repetitive body movements often caused by any one of a wide variety of prescription medications, including some commonly prescribed antidepressants and antipsychotic drugs

temporomandibular joint dysfunction, or jaw pain (TMJ), pain and problems with the alignment and mobility of the jaw

therapeutic nihilism, a disbelief in the effectiveness or value of treatments or therapies, such as drugs and medicines

Tourette syndrome, (repeated, uncontrollable movements or involuntary vocal sounds)

urinary incontinence, refers to the inability to control when urination occurs

vertigo, vertigo is a spinning sensation and can occur even when you are perfectly still.

Western medicine, the type of medical treatment popular in North America and Western European countries based primarily on the use if pharmaceutical drugs and surgery. This is also referred to as "traditional Western medicine. Other types of treatment are referred to as "alternative medicine" or "complementary medicine".

whiplash, an injury to the neck resulting from rapid acceleration or deceleration - as in an automobile accident

Resources

Information on all the resources and references used in this book are available online at the publisher's website http://OldTownPublishing.com

www.ingramcontent.com/pod-product-compliance
Lightning Source LLC
Chambersburg PA
CBHW071433180526
45170CB00001B/323